THE IMMUNE
SYSTEM
CURE

Nature's Way to Super-Powered Health

THE IMMUNE
SYSTEM
CURE

Nature's Way to Super-Powered Health

Lorna R. Vanderhaeghe &
Patrick J. D. Bouic, Ph.D.

VIKING
CANADA

VIKING CANADA

Published by the Penguin Group

Penguin Books, a division of Pearson Canada, 10 Alcorn Avenue, Toronto, Ontario, Canada M4V 3B2

Penguin Books Ltd, 80 Strand, London WC2R 0RL, England

Penguin Putnam Inc., 375 Hudson Street, New York, New York 10014, U.S.A.

Penguin Books Australia Ltd, 250 Camberwell Road, Camberwell, Victoria 3124, Australia

Penguin Books India (P) Ltd, 11, Community Centre, Panchsheel Park, New Delhi – 110 017, India

Penguin Books (NZ) Ltd, cnr Rosedale and Airborne Roads, Albany, Auckland 1310, New Zealand

Penguin Books (South Africa) (Pty) Ltd, 24 Sturdee Avenue, Rosebank 2196, South Africa

Penguin Books Ltd, Registered Offices: 80 Strand, London WC2R 0RL, England

First published in Prentice Hall Canada by Pearson PTR Canada, 1999

Published in Viking Canada by Penguin Books, a division of Pearson Canada, 2002

9 10 WC 03 02

Printed and bound in Canada.

This publication contains the opinions and ideas of its authors and is designed to provide useful
advice in regard to the subject matter covered. The authors and publisher are not engaged in rendering
medical, therapeutic, or other professional services in this publication. This publication is not intended to
provide a basis for action in particular circumstances without consideration by a competent professional.
The authors and publisher expressly disclaim any responsibility for any liability, loss, or risk, personal
or otherwise, which is incurred as a consequence, directly or indirectly, of the use and application of any
of the contents of this book.

NATIONAL LIBRARY OF CANADA CATALOGUING IN PUBLICATION DATA

Vanderhaeghe, Lorna R.
   The immune system cure : nature's way to super-powered health / Lorna R. Vanderhaeghe and
      Patrick J.D. Bouic.

Includes bibliographical references and index.
ISBN 0-670-04395-8

1. Immunity—Popular works. 2. Immunity—Nutritional aspects. 3. Natural immunity.
4. Naturopathy. I. Bouic, Patrick J. D. II. Title.

QR181.7.V36 2002   616.07'9   C2002-905558-X

ATTENTION: CORPORATIONS
Books are available at quantity discounts with bulk purchase for educational, business, or sales promotional
use. For information, please email or write to: Penguin Books, 10 Alcorn Avenue, Suite 304, M4V 3B2.
Email: lorraine.kelly@penguin.ca. Please supply: title of book, ISBN, quantity, how the book will be
used, date needed.

Visit Penguin Books' website at **www.penguin.ca**

This book is dedicated to the health of our children and yours.
For Caitlyn, Kevin, Kyle, Crystal and Marie
and Isabelle

CONTENTS

_____

Acknowledgments

Many people have provided the encouragement, enthusiasm and support to succeed in this project. To my children, Crystal, Kevin, Caitlyn and Kyle, thank you for the hours of patience while I was researching and writing this book. I am deeply grateful for your love and understanding. Mom, thank you for providing me with a strong genetic constitution and the drive to succeed. I am grateful to John Barson for all the back rubs and Internet searches to compile the list of on-line resources. Special regards to Emanuel Cheraskin, MD, DMD, for encouraging me to soar. Rose and Abram Hoffer, thank you for all your encouragement when I worked and studied at the *Journal of Orthomolecular Medicine*. My thanks go to the late Linus Pauling, Ph.D. for sharing with me stories of his wife's determination to succeed in a time when women were not given the recognition they deserved; he inspired me to defy conventional doctrine. Thank you to Siegfried Gursche and Claire Farr for always believing in me. I am grateful to John Morgenthaler for his kindred spirit and respect, and to Ronald Reichert, ND, Udo Erasmus, Ph.D. and Richard Johnson, MD, for the hours of discussion regarding human biochemistry and nutrition. Thank you to my dear friend Josef Tyls, Ph.D. for his research on our water supply and oxidative therapies; to Deane Parkes for his long friendship and continued support on this project; to my staff Hazel Gill and Tanja Hutter for supporting all the efforts required to compile and write this book; and to Andrew Munaweera for his contribution on diabetes; and Ryan Ligeza for his artwork. My thanks go to Lu Cormier for producing this book in record time; to Jim MacLachlan for his editorial advice; and to Liba Berry for her expert editing skills and kind manner. To Dean Hanneford, thank you for pushing all publishing boundaries. I am grateful to David Chapman and Poon Liebenberg for sending me to South Africa to do research for this book. To Mr. Roelof Liebenberg for sharing his life's work with me; and to Patrick for his expertise in immunology, his research and the camaraderie we have shared.

Special thanks go to the pioneers who broke new ground enabling us to provide the latest information to those who are sick and in need. To those whose research and concepts we are sharing with the world, thank you.

Lorna R. Vanderhaeghe

Preface

For decades we have been searching for a cure for cancer, arthritis, the common cold and now AIDS. A magic drug, antibiotic or vaccine have been the focus of this research. Yet we have the most powerful curing machine hardwired into our body—the immune system. Nature eloquently designed the human body with the tools needed to prevent and fight most disease. It is only through neglect, abuse and overuse that we have altered the ability of the immune system to function optimally. This book is not about a magic cure; it is about treatments that boost and balance the immune system to give it the support it needs.

Plenty of solid, current research backs up the many immune enhancers mentioned throughout this book. We hope this quells the constant questions from skeptical physicians and laypeople. Part A provides the foundation of the immune system cure. By adopting the measures presented in chapters 1 to 6, you will ensure peak immunity and maximum protection from disease. Immunology buffs will enjoy chapter 2, and those who are less inclined can use it as a cross-reference for the conditions mentioned in Part B.

Part B focuses on specific diseases that commonly plague our society. Treatment plans are simple, affordable and effective. Discuss the recommendations contained in chapters 7 to 12 with your health care professional and work together to achieve an immune system cure.

Refer to the appendices for useful information about products and resources.

As we enter the new millennium, nothing will be as important to our health as adjusting our lifestyle and maximizing our immunity. Protect yourself and nourish your immune system, and your body's ability to heal will soar.

The History of Medicine

_____

2000 BC
Here, eat this root.

1000 BC
That root is heathen. Here, say this prayer.

1805 AD
That prayer is superstition. Here, drink this potion.

1940 AD
That potion is snake oil. Here, swallow this pill.

1985 AD
That pill is ineffective. Here, take this antibiotic.

2000 AD
That antibiotic doesn't work anymore. Here, eat this root....

—Unknown

Introduction

It is astounding how many people are afflicted by cancer, autoimmune and other degenerative diseases. While genetics and heredity are frequently seen as the culprits, we must also take into account the wear and tear the human immune system sustains as a result of poor nutrition, stress and an unhealthy lifestyle. The key to combatting disease is to ensure the health of the body's immune system, and to recognize that nature has all the answers, in what we call the immune system cure.

Nutrition plays a major role in the prevention of disease. One has only to look at countries like Africa, where malnutrition is rife and the incidence of cancers, parasitic infections, and chronic viral and bacterial conditions are high, to understand the vital role nutrition plays in disease prevention. Few conventional practitioners, however, are willing to consider nutritional deficiencies when treating patients.

The immune system is an integrated network of cells that protect the host in times of an infection. It is a remarkable system in that it is finely tuned to be able to respond quickly in times of need, but it is also a system with many control mechanisms. Should these regulatory mechanisms fail, the response goes uncontrolled and becomes the host's enemy. The immune system turns on itself and destroys healthy cells and tissues or even fails in the face of a viral or bacterial onslaught. Why does this happen? Many reasons can be provided to this question: the most important is that the immune system has to be protected by being fed the correct foods. Second, the stress—physical, emotional and psychological—that we are subjected to each day affects the immune system negatively. When we do not provide the body with the right foods and supplements to combat this onslaught, its resistance starts to fail: the body's natural ability to fight disease diminishes and the possibility of developing degenerative disorders and allergies becomes very real.

This book will help you help your immune system to function optimally. It will discuss the many nutrients (see chapter 3) that are extremely important in providing the immune system the correct substances to react in times of invasion by foreign organisms, but then to return to rest when protective reactions are not required. Good nutrition provides the safety valve to ensure that the immune system does not go on relentlessly in the absence of external stimuli, as is the case in autoimmune disorders (see chapter 9) and allergies (see chapter 10). The safety valve also guarantees the ability of the defense system to seek out cancer cells and to destroy them before they have time to develop into tumors.

Nature does provide us with all the tools to optimize the functioning and health of the immune system. Plant substances are daily being recognized as powerful factors in the fight against disease. We believe that one particularly important phytonutrient complex that includes sterols and sterolins will be the nutrient of the millennium. Sterols and sterolins (a mixture known as Sterinol™) have been shown to have important immune-enhancing effects in helping to maintain a healthy immune system and to guarantee that the cells of this complicated system react efficiently when they are required to. The Sterinol complex ensures that the cells which fight off organisms that tend to live inside our own cells (viruses, parasites and bacteria) are activated and kill off the offending organisms.

One must think of the role played by sterols and sterolins as one of controlling the functions of the immune response, like a seesaw that is capable of "overshooting" when the balance between positive and negative forces are out of tilt. Let us imagine that the positive forces are represented by the "good" regulatory factors secreted by the specialized white blood cells. These forces can only neutralize the "bad" factors when they can be made and released. With viral diseases and bacteria that live inside human cells, unfortunately, these "good" forces are somewhat deficient, especially when the host is malnourished or not providing the body with the right foods. The "bad" factors overpower the failing protective arm and the infection is able to go on uncontrolled. Sterols and sterolins provide the body with the extra weight to balance out this discrepancy. The plant fats provide the cells of the immune response the correct messages to tilt the seesaw into the protective mode, thereby clearing the body of the offending organism.

Sterols and sterolins also regulate or modify the immune response when it is overactive. This is the scenario in chronic degenerative conditions such as rheumatoid arthritis, lupus, and scleroderma, amongst the autoimmune diseases. Also, the same immune dysregulation exists in cases of allergies, including asthma, eczema, dermatitis, sinusitis and rhinitis. Now, due to the increased secretion of the "regulatory" factors, these disorders can be rectified quickly and effectively by sterols and sterolins. The scientific studies presented in this book support this fact.

The immune system cure we recommend in this book is unique in that, unlike traditional therapies, we are not simply treating the patient with drugs that "switch" off the whole response when it is overactive. With Sterinol, we target the cells of the immune system and get them to function normally once again. The immune system cure is not the so-called "shot gun approach" adopted when faced with an immune response that is uncontrolled. Rather, it targets the abnormality and rectifies the fault, without the side effects and toxicity usually associated with drugs acting on the immune system. For the first time, such molecules are able to profoundly and safely modify underlying immune malfunctions and also maintain a healthy natural resistance to infections.

You have at your fingertips the immune system cure. Nature provides it; you have but to make the choice.

—Patrick J.D. Bouic, Ph.D.

Ode to Great Men

In Roelof Liebenberg, I saw a potent spirit,
As powerful as other great men I have been privileged to know:
The late Linus Pauling,
Dr. Emanuel Cheraskin,
Dr. Abram Hoffer;
Men with vision greater than most can ever dream;
Men active and enthusiastic well into their senior years,
Still working, spawning research,
Still striving to help and heal humanity.
These men are my mentors,
Younger in energy than men half their age,
They are gentle giants in their own right;
They inspire us never to give up,
Always to seek out our dreams.

—Lorna R. Vanderhaeghe

Part A

NUTRITION AND THE IMMUNE SYSTEM

1

OUT OF AFRICA

Whatever the mind of man can conceive and believe, he can achieve.

—Napolean Hill

What causes one person to catch a cold or the flu and another to avoid it? What causes one person with HIV never to contract full-blown AIDS and another to succumb and die? Why, with serious outbreaks of infectious diseases, are only a certain number stricken, and of those, why do only some people die? Each individual's lifestyle choices, the foods they eat and the genes their parents gave them is the answer. We can't choose our parents but we can control what we eat and where and how we live.

Virulent new killers, including flesh-eating disease and Ebola virus, are now diseases we are fearful of. Air travel has made it very simple for a virus or bacteria found in one part of the world to be transported along with its host to another. So how do we protect ourselves? Do we don face masks and limit our exposure to people? The solution is much less drastic. The solution, in fact, resides not in some external approach, but within ourselves. Simply giving your immune system the tools to fend off invaders is the answer.

The body's ability to protect itself from offending organisms can be enhanced or weakened by a number of factors. We have each experienced a cold that sets in after an extraordinarily stressful event: too many days of celebration, unrelenting stress or packing too many things into a day without enough sleep can all cause illness. After such traumas as the death of a loved one, a divorce or the loss of a job, those affected are much more susceptible to heart attack, debilitating illness or even cancer. Diet, nutritional supplements, phytonutrients (plant nutrients) and exercise all have a powerful impact on how quickly we recover.

Emotions are deeply linked to the body's immunity. Indeed, joy and fulfillment are potent immune protectors. Loving relationships and the power of prayer cannot be understated in our overall health. Do not dismiss those reports of diseases cured by laughter or prayer. The human nervous system is hardwired to our immunity and researchers are marveling at this fact. So new to the understanding of human physiology are these findings that medical textbooks are being rewritten. Fascinating research will be uncovered in the next decade that will change the way we view our emotions.

Acquired immunodeficiency syndrome (AIDS) and human immuno-deficiency virus (HIV) have done to immunology what understanding the effects of the emotions on human health is doing to the study of neurology. Intense research into the intricacies of the AIDS virus has sent the study of how the body protects us from disease into hyper drive. No other illness has driven researchers so hard to find a cure. The ultimate threat of viruses to human survival became very apparent with the discovery of the HI virus. Fear of this continually mutating virus runs deep. Newspapers are filled daily with reports of more people infected and more deaths. Along with cancer, more money is poured into AIDS research than for any other disease of our day. Scientists are frantically working on finding cures. Each research group wants to be the first to discover a vaccine to prevent cancers or a new antiviral pharmaceutical to kill AIDS.

PLANTS TO THE RESCUE

Many have speculated that due to the sheer number of people affected by AIDS in Africa, the breakthrough in the treatment of this disease would originate there. What no one would have suspected is that this treatment would come from the healing substances found in plants.

Plants not only offer us vitamins, minerals and trace elements, they also provide phytonutrients (*phyto*=plant) that are found in plants to protect the plant from its environmental predators: sun damage, pests and toxins. Common drugs have been synthesized from plants: digoxin was originally derived from foxglove and aspirin from willow bark. Before the advent of pharmaceuticals, traditional healers used plants in their repertoire of treatments. Forgotten once antibiotics came into use, plants are now being revitalized as a treatment approach because bacteria have become resistant to antibiotic therapy. Standard drug therapies have been less than effective in treating 20th century diseases caused by poor nutrition, stress and environmental toxins. Natural medicines, used for generations, have the ability to stimulate the human immune system to fight its own battles.

The immune system is the benefactor of plant nutrients in that phytonutrients have the ability to enhance the body's self-protective powers. Plant constituents known as sterols and sterolins help the immune system to stop cancer, kill bacteria, destroy viruses or slow the aging process. Africa is the country that gives us the sterolin-specific product that enhances the way our immune system works.

Although there are many immune-enhancing nutrients and foods, none has the immune-enhancing effects of a unique product out of Africa called Moducare® Sterinol™. Developed from plant sources, this combination of sterols and sterolins has been shown to have powerful healing effects on cancer, AIDS, tuberculosis, and autoimmune disorders.

The story of how a sterol/sterinol-based remedy came about begins with one man, Mr. Roelof Wilke Liebenburg; we will call him R.W. His inquisitive mind allowed him to see what others could not, and his determination to find the answers would not let him quit. A soft-spoken South African gentleman, R.W. knew that he was on the track of an important discovery, a cure for cancer. This is his story.

As a boy, R.W. lived in a remote area of South Africa where a doctor was a luxury beyond the means of a poor family. His mother was known far and wide for having a folk remedy for whatever ailed you. She nursed her family, friends and neighbors through colds, flus, fevers, infections and childhood diseases with many homemade brews. His mother's use of nature to heal left a lasting impression on R.W., and years later the healing ability of plants would become invaluable to his life's work.

In 1958, R.W.'s quest began. One of his relatives, Oom Koos, a 76-year-old man, was discharged from a hospital in Pretoria with prostate cancer. Doctors told the family that the cancer was too advanced for surgery and there was no other treatment available. Oom Koos was already slipping in and out of coma and was expected to live only a few more days. Relatives gathered and friends called to pay their last respects. One neighbor, on hearing that the old gentleman was suffering from "old man's gland disease," went out and dug up a wild plant growing in a nearby veldt and told Mr. Koos's wife how to prepare and administer a traditional folk remedy for her husband's condition. Within a week, Mr. Koos was sitting up in bed and asking for food. He lived another 10 years and died of something unrelated to his cancer.

The experience of Oom Koos, combined with his mother's natural-healing practices and the loss of many friends to cancer, whetted R.W.'s insatiable appetite to find a cure for this most dreaded disease. He read books by the late Dr. Max Gerson, a physician who created a strict fruit and vegetable juice program for cancer patients. Gerson's approach (which is still used today) confirmed R.W.'s belief that plants have properties that will cure cancer. For the next 40 years he examined the plant components that were used to treat Oom Koos's cancer. Even though he had no formal scientific training, R.W. taught himself chemistry, biology and physiology. He read and researched any information he could find on cancer, the immune system and the innate healing ability of the body. He read reports about the cancer-fighting features of certain foods and studied research documents published by the National Cancer Agency in the United States. Realizing there must be important curative properties in all plants, he diligently searched for the clues that would ultimately lead to a potent immune system cure.

Important people who would help him realize his dream entered his life. Through a wonderful young woman, whom he later married, he met Dr. Scheffel, who went to South Africa in the early sixties to research trachoma, a disease of the eyes. Dr. Scheffel was the first medical person to listen to R.W.'s theories. He even went so far as to visit with Oom Koos and drink the traditional healing brew. Dr. Scheffel became a believer and promised to assist R.W. in helping to research this remedy.

Some years later, Dr. Scheffel, now living in Germany, contacted a renowned urologist, Dr. Dieter Ebbinghaus, to discuss the South African prostate remedy. Dr. Ebbinghaus was in charge of the Kreis-krankenhaus, Hellersen-L"udenscheid, a hospital where all the patients from a large area of Germany were sent for treatment of their prostate problems. After Dr. Ebbinghaus studied the reports about the prostate remedy, he agreed to do a small study on his patients. He treated his patients for one month, monitoring them closely for any adverse effects. Dr. Ebbinghaus's findings were encouraging: certain symptoms of a severe prostate problem in men called benign prostatic hypertrophy (BPH) were reduced—urine flow was increased, residual urine measured in the bladder had decreased and the muscle tone of the bladder, already stretched because of chronic urine retention, was also improved. Clearly, this plant extract could be effective, and the research continued.

In the meantime, R.W. had met Karl Pegel, who was studying phytochemistry (the chemistry of plants), at the University of the Witwaterstrand, Johannesburg. Pegel completed his studies and became a professor. R.W. asked Dr. Pegel to isolate and identify the active compound in the plant being used for prostate problems. Pegel agreed, and for a small amount of money R.W. sponsored research assistant Engela de Witt to help Pegel isolate the compound. After some months, de Witt extracted a fatty substance from the plant, which was then sent to the Council for Scientific and Industrial Research, South Africa, for structure determination. R.W. also took some of the mixture and filled 300 capsules with 10 milligrams each. With these 300 capsules he flew to Dusseldorf to meet with Dr. Scheffel and Dr. Ebbinghaus.

Dr. Ebbinghaus took the capsules and started treating patients with the mixture. He found this isolated ingredient did not work as well as the first substance, but it still had a healing effect. In the meantime, the fatty substance was identified as sitosterol. R.W. was disappointed because sitosterol had been identified in 1922, and the U.S. Cancer Agency had found it ineffective in the treatment of cancer. But Dr. Pegel knew plant chemistry and he recognized something they had been missing.

Pegel knew that there are bound and free sterols in plants called sterols and sterolins. Sterolin is a sterol molecule that has attached itself to a glucose molecule. He realized that due to its structure, the sterolin would be absorbed better than the sterol molecule because it is more soluble. During the process to isolate the active ingredient of the plant, the sterols and sterolins had been removed from the plant by hydrolysis. This process breaks off the glucose molecules, yielding only sterols and no sterolins. The breakthrough came when the research team realized that, ideally, sterols and sterolins had to be in as close a form to nature as possible. This was the reason the isolated substance that was used on Dr. Ebbinghaus's patients did not work as well. It was missing the most important ingredient—the sterolin, the key to the immune-enhancing effect. (Researchers often strive to have a plant substance so isolated that they miss out on many other important healing aspects of the whole plant. This is so with beta-carotene. Many researchers believe that all the different carotenoids should be taken together and that by consuming only the isolated ingredient we are limiting their effects.)

Professor Rogers then joined the research team to develop a product that had the same properties as the plant used in the traditional remedy. A product was developed and capsules were sent to Dr. Ebbinghaus in Germany.

Several clinical trials were performed there, resulting in the release of a patented remedy in 1974 for benign prostatic hypertrophy (BPH). After 25 years, this special combination of sterols and sterolins is still the market leader for the treatment of BPH in Germany. Due to the country's strict medical control regulations, the original formulation has not been altered. Further research and advanced technology in product manufacture resulted in an improved product called Moducare® Sterinol™ (we will refer to it here as Sterinol).

EXCITING RESEARCH

The initial breakthrough which showed the effectiveness of sterols and sterolins in treating benign prostatic hypertrophy (BPH) was followed by further research and clinical trials. These tests showed that although Sterinol did not offer a magical cure for every ailment tested for, a majority of patients tested experienced improvement shortly after taking it. Finally, after 40 years of research and development, the Sterinol combination became available for over-the-counter sale in South Africa as Moducare.

With the product on the open market, an overwhelmingly positive response came from medical doctors and pharmacists. Autoimmune disorders (especially rheumatoid arthritis), prostate problems, cancer, herpes, asthma, HIV and AIDS, stress-induced illness and diabetes are just a few of the disorders that were benefitting from Sterinol.

After overcoming more problems than the Imax team encountered on Mount Everest, R.W. Liebenburg's dream was realized. The world's first nontoxic remedy that enables the human body to win its own battles against disease was available. But it was not enough for R.W. to find an immune system cure; he also insisted that it be proven beyond a shadow of a doubt that the remedy truly worked. To this end, his team of researchers at the University of Stellenbosch, Cape Town, South Africa, continue to carry out double-blind, placebo-controlled trials to prove the effectiveness of Sterinol.

Although Sterinol is a remarkable product with remarkable healing capabilities, we do not believe that one product alone can cure all ailments. A supportive approach to healing must be adopted, and the benefits of good nutrition cannot be understated. Combine the many recommendations we put forth in this book and you will increase your life span and live in excellent health.

2

UNDERSTANDING IMMUNITY

We command Nature only by obeying her.

—Francis Bacon

The immune system is a highly specialized front-line defense that identifies, remembers, attacks and destroys disease-causing invaders and transformed or infected cells. Essentially, the immune system is the body's means of surveillance, intended to protect it from disease by searching out and destroying any health-damaging agents. When functioning optimally, the immune system is a powerful protector. Few viruses, bacteria, fungi or parasites are allowed to set up house and wreak havoc if the immune system is operating at peak performance. The immune system is so determined to annihilate invaders that it can often go awry and begin to damage the body itself, as happens in diseases such as lupus and rheumatoid arthritis.

To appreciate how indispensable the immune system is, we need only consider the fate of those with inherited or acquired immune deficiency syndromes. Infants born with defective immune systems can only survive in a completely sterile environment free of microorganisms that cause infection. People whose immune systems have been artificially suppressed by drugs, to prevent rejection of transplant organs, are temporarily highly susceptible to infections and certain cancers. The same is true for cancer patients undergoing treatments such as bone marrow transplants. An immune system suppressed or destroyed is vulnerable to attack.

Acquired immunodeficiency syndrome (AIDS) has brought the field of immunology to center stage. Never before in the history of medicine has a disease been so resistant to human endeavors to find a cure. People with AIDS are infected with the human immunodeficiency virus (HIV), which impairs the immune system, thus making those infected highly susceptible to opportunistic infections such as pneumonia. As a result, minor infections, which a healthy immune system would be able to deal with, can have a devastating, and often fatal, effect.

How Do You Know if Your Immune System Is Dysfunctional?

- frequent colds and flu
- herpes (cold sore) outbreaks
- allergies
- continual fatigue
- candida yeast overgrowth
- painful joints and muscles
- parasite infections
- psoriasis and eczema
- inflammatory disorders

Immunology, the study of the immune system, arose out of the observation that people who have contracted and recovered from infections such as mumps, chicken pox or measles, rarely, if ever, get the same disease again. With this protective immunity, an individual enjoys specific and long-lasting protection against contracting the same disease again. Childhood diseases are a kind of training ground for the immune system, whereby it learns to defend itself properly from invading organisms.

Immunity involves the production of a specific protein called an antibody. Antibodies are designed to destroy a particular invader called an antigen. Antigens are foreign substances that can cause the immune system to respond. They reside on the surface of bacteria or viruses as locator codes in the form of proteins and polysaccharides. If a specific antigen invades the body, an antibody will be produced to destroy that particular antigen and only that antigen. If a different type of antigen is presented, the same process occurs, whereby an antibody specific to that antigen will be produced and so on, over and over again. The ability to ward off disease through our defenses is called resistance, and this specific resistance to disease due to the presence of antigen-specific antibodies is called immunity. The body also offers nonspecific resistance to disease through other defense mechanisms.

IMMUNITY WE ARE BORN WITH

Nonspecific immunity or resistance to disease is inherited in healthy individuals and provides a general response against a wide variety of foreign invaders. Included in the defense mechanisms are the skin and mucus membranes. Most of us would not consider the skin as part of the immune system, but if intact, it is an impenetrable barrier and the first line of defense against invaders. Mucus membranes, lining body cavities that are open to the outside world and potential invaders, are also important to defense. Saliva, tears and vaginal secretions are other protectors, diluting and washing microbes away.

Phagocytes

If a lucky invader actually finds its way into the body, another method of destruction devised by the immune system is phagocytosis, which means eating and digesting foreign matter. The cells involved in phagocytosis, called phagocytes include granulocytes and macrophages. We will learn more about macrophages later. When infection occurs, phagocytes rush to the area to digest and destroy. Since they don't have receptors like other immune cells, their effectiveness at destroying viruses, bacteria, old and dead cells is wide-ranging. Although not all invaders are destroyed, this method is quite effective. Staphylococci, tubercle bacillus and other microbes often destroy the phagocyte or remain dormant for months or even years just waiting for the immune system to become weak and susceptible to attack. If the immune system is in optimal condition, however, these troublemakers can be dealt with or kept silent as long as we live.

Fever

Fever is another method the body uses to defend us from bacteria and viruses. A high body temperature slows down invaders and can even kill them. Pyrogens released from phagocytes cause fever to be induced.

Inflammation

Inflammation is another way the body defends itself. Within seconds of an injury or invasion, the immune system is activated. Redness, pain, swelling and heat are all active protective responses to dispose of microbes, toxins or any other foreign material at the site of inflammation. This process also prepares the site for repair and prevents further damage.

Complement

Another immune agent called complement is a combination of eleven protein enzymes that circulate in the blood and act as catalysts in antibody reactions. When an invader appears, complement releases its first enzyme; then each enzyme in a cascade is released until all eleven enzymes are used up. Each reaction has a particular function in killing invaders. Complement proteins attract phagocytes to the site of inflammation and cause them to be very voracious eaters.

Natural Killer Cells

Natural killer cells (NK cells) are the body's first line of defense against invading microorganisms, parasites, viruses, bacteria and fungi. As well, these cells also seek out and destroy on contact cancer cells before they find a place to attach and develop into a tumor. Natural killer cells, like phagocytes, do not need to be told to deal with an invader or infected cell. They act on their own. Unlike other cells of the immune system, NK cells do not have memory, which means they have to deal with each invader as if it was seen for the first time.

Natural killer cells have some properties similar to cytotoxic T-cells in that they kill by releasing toxic enzymes that destroy the invader. NK cells, however, are more voracious killers than cytotoxic T-cells. NK cells provide the first line of attack against cancer cells and cells infected by pathogens other than viruses. Research shows that NK cells are reduced in number in cancer patients and the reduction is associated with the severity of the cancer.

NK cells do not need permission from a T4 cell (helper T-cell) and are free to attack. Of particular interest is the ability of NK cells to release interferons that stop viruses from replicating. These interferons also improve the killing ability of NK cells, making them more aggressive and calling more NK cells to arms.

THE GUARDIANS OF YOUR IMMUNE SYSTEM

Some invading organisms are so determined to get through the physical barriers provided by our innate immunity and past phagocytes that these barriers are not enough to defend the body from disease. This is especially true if, due to poor nutrition and excessive stress, the immune system is not functioning optimally. This highly evolved system has all the properties to defeat disease and keep us healthy. All we have to do is provide it with the appropriate tools to do its job: good nutrition, food supplements, stress reducers and exercise. The nutritional supplements, dietary factors and lifestyle choices important for the immune system will be described in subsequent chapters.

The immune system's primary role is to fight disease. A quick review of certain aspects of immunity will explain what a finely tuned instrument the human body is.

The **thymus** is a flat, soft, pinkish-gray gland in the upper chest in front of the heart. Relatively large in the newborn (about the size of the baby's heart), it continues to grow up to the age of puberty, when it weighs about 1.2 ounces.

T-cells are matured in the thymus, which gives them the specific structures needed for fighting foreign organisms. The T-cells then migrate into the lymphatic system.

The **lymphatic system** is made up of lymph fluid, lymphatic vessels, bone marrow (this is where immune cells are derived) lymph nodes, spleen and tonsils. It plays a role in the elimination of toxic waste from tissues and is an integral part of the immune system. Fluid is pumped through this system via the muscles, not the heart. A sluggish lymphatic system is most often due to a lack of exercise. When the body is fighting off an infection, the lymph glands become swollen with the additional burden of trying to clear and clean the system.

B-cells develop in the bone marrow. They are not affected by the thymus, but are modified by certain T-cells. They reside in lymph nodes.

The immune response is like a well-trained orchestra with the thymus at center stage. At birth, the thymus, located behind the breastbone, is bigger than your heart. (Physicians in the early part of the 20th century unknowingly thought that a large thymus was a defect in infants and radiated the thymus in order to shrink it.) As we age, the thymus slowly shrinks, causing a subsequent decline in immunity. Until recently this shrinkage was thought to be a normal aspect of aging, which caused the production of thymulin, a hormone the thymus secretes which causes the production of T-cells to be reduced and the immune system to fail to mature. Without mature T-cells, B-cells are unable to make antibodies, resulting in an increase in infections, cancer and autoimmune disorders. It is now known that shrinkage of the thymus is not inevitable and we will show you that it is even reversible.

Immune Cells

Our blood contains both red cells and white cells. The white cells are the immune cells. One type of white blood cell, the lymphocytes, are born in the marrow of the long bones of the body. They are long-lived cells that carry memory of past infections. As lymphocytes mature, some remain in the marrow and develop into B-cells, and others spread throughout the body via the blood, to the lymph, and go to the thymus gland, where they become T-cells. In the thymus, each T-cell is taught to recognize only one of millions of antigens. T-cells only recognize one specific antigen. In our environment, the immune system encounters millions of antigens, but only one specific T-cell will respond to each individual antigen.

T-cells are also taught to recognize the difference between invading cells ("non-self") and our own cells ("self"). Normally, the immune system attacks only substances or pathogens that are thought of as foreigners. They may be invaders from outside the body, or cancer cells made within the body. However, sometimes the immune system may be confused and attack healthy body cells.

It is possible that certain infectious organisms may have a role in confusing the immune system. Sexually transmitted chlamydia and streptoccous bacteria may be implicated in causing the immune system to turn upon itself. When this happens, autoimmune disorders occur (see chapter 9). Such diseases (for example, rheumatoid arthritis, lupus, and pernicious anemias, among others) arise in response to an overproduction of lymphokines which promote the B-cells to make antibodies. Those antibodies then attack the body and the cycle continues. Certain phytonutrients, the sterols and sterolins, cause the T-cells to release the correct lymphokines to correct the immune system and restore health.

Cytokines are proteins secreted by monocytes called monokines and lymphocytes called lymphokines that regulate the magnitude of an inflammatory or immune response.

IMMUNE SYSTEM WARRIORS

T-cells are responsible for cell-mediated responses to disease. Cell-mediated immunity is very important in fighting viruses, fungi, yeast, bacteria and parasites, especially those that reside within cells. It causes immune cells to travel throughout the body on a seek-and-destroy mission. They then lock onto cells and destroy them.

There are three main types of T-cells: helper T-cells, cytotoxic T-cells and suppressor T-cells.

Helper T-cells

Helper T-cells, also known as T4 cells or CD4 cells, sound the emergency alarm and assist the cytotoxic T-cells in their action. They also secrete interleukin-2 (IL-2) that stimulates the growth, abundance and killing ability of cytotoxic T-cells. Helper T-cells also secrete proteins that increase the inflammatory response and the ability of macrophages (a large white blood cell that arrives at the site of inflammation) to kill. Without permission from the helper T-cells, other immune cells and cytotoxic T-cells cannot do their job. Helper T-cells also tell B-cells to produce antibodies.

Helper T-cells can be further differentiated into T_H1 and T_H2. These two types of helper cells produce very different lymphokines. T_H1 and T_H2 must be in balance; an overabundance of one or deficiency of another causes disease. When T_H1 and T_H2 are in balance, health is maintained. (At the end of this chapter we will examine how Sterinol promotes this balance.)

T_H1 cells produce lymphokines that enhance the ability of the immune system to respond to virus, intracellular bacteria, fungi or parasites and activate cytotoxic or suppressor T-cells. These cells kill abnormal cells infected with bacteria, viruses and cancer. T$_H$1 cells also control the activity of T$_H$2 cells. Sterinol increases T$_H$1 and therefore promotes a positive immune response.

T$_H$2 cells function more in relation to allergic reactions or antibody responses. T$_H$2-mediated responses increase antibody production and when out of balance can cause destruction of cells of the "self." T$_H$2 releases IL6, a powerful interleukin involved in inflammatory processes seen in rheumatoid arthritis. The ultimate immune modulating product would increase levels of T$_H$1 and down-regulate the release of IL6 from T$_H$2 cells. Past and current research at the University of Stellenbosch, in Cape Town, South Africa, is focusing on ways to increase or promote T$_H$1 production using Sterinol.

Cytotoxic T-cells

Cytotoxic T-cells, also called Killer T-cells (we will call them cytotoxic in order not to confuse you with natural Killer cells) travel to the site of invasion, where they attach to malignant (cancerous) cells or infected cells. Cytotoxic T-cells also have specialized surface receptors that can recognize specific antigens. They then inject a cytokine that destroys the antigen directly. They also release a factor that improves the eating and digesting activity of macrophages, attracts more macrophages to the site and encourages the macrophages to stay at the site of infection. Most important, cytotoxic T-cells also secrete interferons, which stop viruses from reproducing and enhance the killing action of the T-cells themselves. Cytotoxic T-cells are especially effective against cancer cells and slow-growing bacteria such as tuberculosis.

Suppressor T-cells

Suppressor T-cells shut down certain activities of the immune response several weeks after an infection. They help maintain a balance in the immune system until another invader arrives. Suppressor T-cells also stop cytotoxic T-cells from releasing cytokines and also stop the production of antibodies. A normal ratio of helper T-cells to suppressor T-cells is 2 to 1. When suppressor cells are reduced, B-cells are left to continue their function unregulated and wreak havoc in the body.

Cells of the Immune System

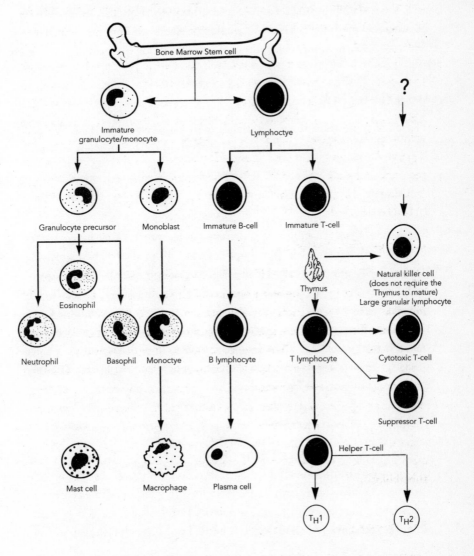

Every day, thousands of microscopic reactions occur swiftly and accurately before any symptoms of illness occur. Billions of T-cells communicate to keep us functioning optimally.

Some of the immune cells secrete the cytokines or immuno-regulating factors interferon and interleukins. Cytokines are proteins with very important immune functions. Two types of cytokines include lymphokines, produced by lymphocytes, and monokines, produced by monocytes. Immune cells have the ability to recognize and bind with these cytokines. These biochemical messengers have many different effects on immune cells. Every day new cytokines and their unique actions are being discovered.

Interleukins

There are more than thirty interleukins (IL) discovered to date. We will discuss the following: interleukin-1, interleukin-2, interleukin-4 and interleukin-6.

Interleukin-1

Interleukin-1 is a cytokine that is involved in the process that induces fever and, as discussed earlier in the chapter, fever kills or slows down a virus or bacteria. Even a temperature rise of 2 to 3 degrees can be enough to accomplish the task. Macrophages produce the most IL-1. Once IL-1 is released, it encourages T-cells to produce more IL-2. By now you understand how interconnected the properties of the immune system are, and you are probably wondering how all of these reactions occur without a glitch. Often, things do go awry, causing allergic reactions, muscle and nerve abnormalities and conditions such as fibromyalgia.

Interleukin-2

Interleukin-2 helps helper T-cells to tell cytotoxic T-cells to destroy an invader. It also informs all T-cells to release more IL-2 as required and therefore be able to destroy more invaders. It is especially effective in enhancing immune responses against tumors. Interleukin-2 is a very powerful immunomodulator which also causes more T-cells to be produced.

Interleukin-4

Interleukin-4 enhances the ability of B-cells to make antibodies (specifically, IgG and IgE, discussed later in the chapter). It also stimulates helper T-cells and cytotoxic T-cells to perform their job. Overproduction of IL-4 promotes allergic responses. Studies that focused on lowering IL-4 show that low levels of IL-4 inhibited IgE antibodies, thus reducing allergic responses.

However, modulators of the immune system should seek a balance, not reduce IL-4 to the point that IgE production by B-cells is inhibited entirely, and cytotoxic T-cell activity is reduced.

Interleukin-6

Interleukin-6 is released by macrophages, monocytes and some T-cells, and induces B-cells to produce antibodies. An abnormal production of IL-6 is associated with autoimmune disorder and inflammatory and allergic conditions. Studies show that psoriasis is associated with T_H2 cells releasing an overabundance of IL-6, which increases the production of skin cells. Research using Sterinol found that supplementation increased T_H1 and down-regulated T_H2, resulting in a decline of IL-6 release and a complete remission of psoriasis symptoms.

An abnormal production of cytokines can lead to serious immune dysregulation and, in certain situations, the production of autoantibodies. Autoantibodies are antibodies that recognize and attack the body's own tissues. In this situation, the body continues to attack itself unregulated; the resulting inflammation is generally specific to certain regions of the body. Some disorders that result from autoantibody production include: rheumatoid arthritis, which affects joints; multiple sclerosis, in which the myelin sheaths surrounding nerves are destroyed; Crohn's disease, whereby the colon cells are attacked; systemic lupus erythematosus, which affects connective tissue; and Type I diabetes mellitus, which involves the pancreas.

Anticancer Warriors

For years scientists have been trying to enhance the immune system to mount an all-out war on cancer. Cytokines such as interleukin-2, interferon and tumor necrosis factor (TNF) have been synthesized and made available as prescription drugs to be used as immunotherapies to treat certain cancers. In very large doses, these cytokines have shown some positive results, especially for Kaposi's sarcoma, hairy-cell leukemia and renal-cell carcinoma. Unfortunately, serious side effects such as bone-marrow suppression, severe weight loss and liver damage also resulted. Nutritional science has taken immunotherapy one step further and found that many natural substances, especially the phytonutrient Sterinol, have the ability to increase the body's own natural production of these cytokines without side effects.

Interferon, the Virus Killer

Interferons are the immune system's front-line defense against most viruses. Several types of interferon exist—gamma, beta and alpha interferon. Interferons cause cells that are not infected with a virus to be resistant to infection. Viruses can only cause disease if they can duplicate themselves within cells. Interferon halts that replication process and is thus a potent virus killer. Interferon is also secreted by T-cells in order to call natural killer cells (NK cells) to battle at the site of infected cells. Although the US Food and Drug Administration (FDA) has approved a synthesized interferon for application in the treatment of hepatitis C and hairy-cell leukemia, results have been disappointing and the side effects severe.

Tumor Necrosis Factor

Tumor necrosis factor (TNF) is released by macrophages and induces fever. It kills some cancer cells and causes the production of lymphokines. As with interferon, scientists have synthesized tumor necrosis factor.

B-cells

The body not only produces thousands of T-cells but also thousands of B-cells, all capable of responding to their own specific antigens. B-cells derive mainly from bone marrow and set up house in the lymph nodes; unlike T-cells, they do not circulate in the blood. Their role is to produce and secrete antibodies. Each B-cell is specific to one particular antigen. B-cells ensure antibody production against antigens with the help of T-cells. They also code for antigens and signal that an antigen is present in order for a T-cell to do its work.

When an invader is present, T-cells tell B-cells to start producing antibodies. B-cells then turn into plasma cells, whereby millions of antibodies specific to the invader cells are produced. Once the antibodies are produced, they are sent into the bloodstream to lock onto an antigen and destroy it. Many antibodies may coat an invader, often completely inactivating it or halting it long enough to mark it for destruction by other immune cells.

Plasma cells memorize the invader's antigens and become memory B-cells. In this way, if another invasion occurs, antibodies will be made available much more rapidly. Plasma cells are relatively short-lived, lasting only 4 to

5 days. During this time, antibodies are secreted at the phenomenal rate of 2,000 molecules per second. The B-cells that do not become plasma cells remain as memory B-cells and live for months or years, ready to forcefully and rapidly take action the next time the same invader appears. Memory cells never forget—they will always remember an antigen that has triggered an immune response.

Antibodies

The five classes of antibodies called immunoglobulins (Ig) include IgA, IgE, IgG, IgM and IgD. We will discuss the first four because IgD is rare and its activity is not clear.

IgA is found in tears, milk, sweat and saliva as well as on mucus membranes. It is involved in holding off invaders or pushing them out of the body. When secretory IgA found in the gastrointestinal tract is low, immune deficiency is common.

IgE is involved in allergic reactions, whereby mast cells (large cells that occur in connective tissues) are encouraged to release histamine (a substance that mediates allergic reactions). In cases of severe allergic reaction, too much histamine causes a system overload that may result in anaphylactic reactions that can result in death. IgE's protective mechanism triggers inflammatory reactions, which help to protect the body against parasite infections. Hay fever and other similar inflammatory responses are thought to be protective, even though sufferers would disagree.

IgG is the most abundant antibody. It coats microorganisms and is specialized to kill certain bacteria and viruses. It also activates a series of enzymes that enhance the digestion of invaders. IgG can punch holes in cell membranes, allowing access to the internal contents of the cell, which is especially important for attacking intracellular viruses. There are four subclasses of IgG, and if even one is low it can impair immune function.

Being of larger size, IgM operates in the bloodstream only and engages in disabling bacteria.

ANATOMY OF A COLD

So what does all this mean for how our bodies respond to an invader or illness? Here is how it all works when a cold virus enters your body. First, a macrophage encounters an intruder. It eats and digests the virus and presents a piece of the invader to a helper T-cell. Now the T-cell jumps onto the macrophage, attaches to it and causes the macrophage to release its messengers to tell other T-cells to look out for the same invaders. At the same time, the T-cell is also activated to tell B-cells to start producing antibodies to recognize the invader.

By now you probably have a runny nose, aches and pains have set in, and you are feeling dreadful. Depending on which virus has invaded your body, it may take a while for your B-cells to produce enough antibodies to fight off the virus. Your temperature has gone up to try to kill off some of the virus as well. You may be halfway through a box of tissues as your immune system tries to eliminate the virus from mucus membranes via your nose. It may take several days for you to feel better depending on the severity of the bug you caught and how primed your immune system was to take action.

When the B-cells have accomplished their job of producing enough antibodies to annihilate the virus, suppressor T-cells come in and tell the B-cells to stop. Your symptoms will soon abate and you will begin to feel well again. If you are infected with the same virus later, your immune system will remember and immediately respond with the appropriate antibodies and you should not develop symptoms. In other words, you will be immune.

Clinical trials using the phytonutrient Sterinol have found that when the helper cells T_H1 and T_H2 are in balance, the body is in a state of good health. When T_H1 drops due to cortisol release, as happens when you are experiencing unrelenting stress, T_H2 increases, and cancer, allergies and autoimmune disorders can appear. Another side effect of T_H2 increase is a reduction in cytotoxic T-cell activity. One capsule of Sterinol three times a day on an empty stomach increased T_H1 dramatically while reducing T_H2. IL-6 was also shut off and the corresponding inflammatory reactions ceased.

An overproduction of IL-6 also causes calcium to be released from bone into the blood. Osteoporosis, a condition caused by poor calcium regulation, is effectively treated using a combination of Sterinol and calcium citrate over the long term. Sterinol switches off IL-6, allowing calcium to stay in bone. Calcium citrate, along with boron and other bone-enhancing minerals, can help to rebuild bone.

Like a person walking a tightrope, the immune system shifts and adjusts to each challenge. Our immune system is programmed for health, and Sterinol is like the bar the tightrope walker carries. It provides the balance.

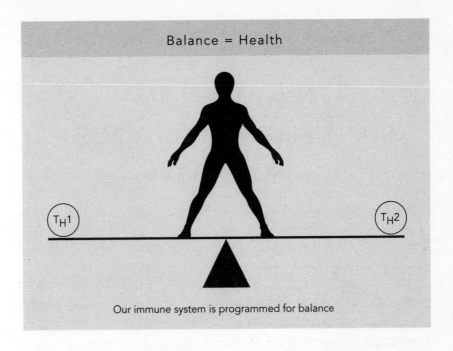

Balance = Health

T_H1 T_H2

Our immune system is programmed for balance

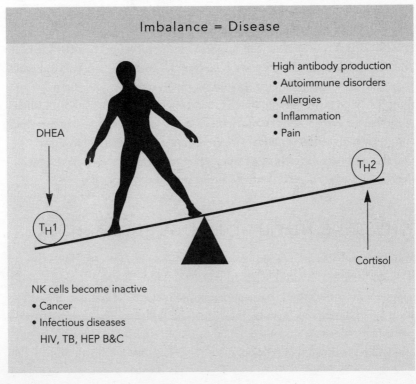

Imbalance = Disease

High antibody production
- Autoimmune disorders
- Allergies
- Inflammation
- Pain

DHEA

T_H2

T_H1

Cortisol

NK cells become inactive
- Cancer
- Infectious diseases
  HIV, TB, HEP B&C

TEN NUTRITIONAL SUPPLEMENTS TO BOOST IMMUNITY

What a piece of work is man! . . . in form and moving, how express and admirable. In action how like an angel!

—William Shakespeare

This book focuses on how to boost or balance the immune system so that it is able it to do what it was designed to do: fight disease and maintain good health. Prevention is the key. Good nutrition and healthy lifestyle choices can give you the protection you need. Moreover, research indicates that nutritional supplements, including phytonutrients and vitamins and minerals, have tremendous immune-enhancing abilities. Follow the guidelines suggested for each of the ten nutrients discussed in this chapter. In less than thirty days you will look and feel more vibrant and energetic. Frequent colds and flus will become a thing of the past, your energy levels will reach new heights and you will have launched your immune system cure.

WHY TAKE NUTRITIONAL SUPPLEMENTS?

You have probably asked it and we have definitely been asked, "Why should we supplement our diets with nutrients?" The answer is simple. Food supplements are exactly that, supplements to the food you eat. If you eat junk food, or are too busy to eat, or are on a weight-loss diet or fitness program, or if you are under stress, you may not be getting adequate nutrients and will require supplementation.

Several problems with the way our food is produced, as well as the way we consume food, have caused the need to supplement our diets with vitamins and minerals: foods that are harvested before they are ripe; foods grown on soils exhausted of their essential elements; eating parts of the plant, not the whole plant; eating refined or highly processed foods that are only fortified with B_1, B_2, B_3 and iron, but not with chromium, manganese, molybdenum, copper or zinc; genetically engineered or hybrid foods that are bred to resist disease in the plants or to retard decay and improve appearance, but not for nutritional content—all contribute to the need for food supplements.

Vitamins and minerals are required as enzymes and coenzymes (which work to facilitate other reactions) for every function in the body. If levels are inadequate, degenerative disorders such as heart disease, arthritis, fatigue, digestive disturbances, infectious and inflammatory diseases will set in. Deficiency of nutrients in the diet also results in food malabsorption syndromes, especially in the elderly. Hypochlorhydria, a reduction in the amount of stomach acid produced, is one such syndrome common in the elderly. It seriously affects nutrient absorption from food and is linked to disease states. Once thought only a problem in the elderly, we now know that it is also found in people whose diets consist largely of packaged and processed foods.

Stress is a part of life and, good or bad, has an impact on our nutrient levels. Stress triggers a biological response during which powerful changes occur: heart rate and blood pressure increase; the adrenal glands are activated; blood sugar levels rise; and the body experiences an increased need for protein. If your nutrient level is low, these natural responses will deplete the body's stores of vitamins and minerals.

Matters are further complicated because even if we eat fresh fish, organic meats and organic fresh produce that has been allowed to vine-ripen, we cannot be guaranteed of every nutrient in the doses required to maintain optimal health. Nature doesn't provide exactly 5 milligrams of zinc in every nut; nutritional content is arbitrary, determined by the weather and the quality of the soil. By choosing organic foods, we can increase our chances of getting the nutrition we need. We all know, however, that most people don't eat 7 to 10 fruits or vegetables daily. For many of us, junk foods and fast food have become a way of life, and even finding the time to eat three meals a day can be difficult.

If you are fortunate enough to eat only organic foods, live in a stress-free environment and have inherited a good genetic makeup, you may be one

What is a Free Radical?

Little was known about free radicals until about 40 years ago. Today they are considered a major component in aging and disease progression. Research has shown that many diseases such as rheumatoid arthritis and cancer are the result of free radical damage in the body.

Free radicals are a natural by-product of everyday reactions that produce energy for the body. The energy is produced by reactions between many substances and oxygen. Without energy production the body cannot survive. Think of the serious impairment to life that chronic fatigue syndrome causes with its malfunctioning energy production.

Molecules including oxygen, fatty acids, amino acids and DNA are the basic components used to build and repair the body. Molecules are held together by electrons. Stable molecules have electrons that are paired. When a molecule does not have a pair, it becomes unstable and reactive. A free radical is that unstable molecule that is highly reactive and searching for a pair to make it stable. It will do anything to find a partner, including stealing and damaging other molecules. If a stable molecule loses an electron, it becomes a free radical, which then steals an electron from another molecule and so on. Stealing an electron from another molecule creates a chain reaction in which thousands of free radicals are released and cause damage and destruction until the reaction is squelched. Think of a tiny spot of rust on the fender of your car. If this tiny spot is left unattended, it will eventually become a big rusty hole. Fortunately, free radical damage can be easily kept in check by using potent antioxidants including vitamin E, vitamin C, selenium and vitamin A.

Exposure to toxins such as tobacco smoke, prescription drugs, environmental pollutants, radiation and even exercise increases free radical reactions in the body. The immune system also produces exorbitant amounts of free radicals as a normal process to destroy invading bacteria and viruses. Free radical production is a process developed by the body to eliminate potential dangerous substances but, left unchecked, free radical damage can do more harm than good. This is where the exciting field of nutrition plays a role.

Destruction of healthy cells can be avoided by simply improving diet and adding nutritional supplements, especially antioxidants and nature's powerful protectors—phytochemicals.

of the few who do not need to take supplements. But for those who want to protect themselves from cancer, it is better to be on the safe side and use nutritional supplements as insurance against disease. Good health is the payout.

TEN IMPORTANT NUTRITIONAL SUPPLEMENTS

- Vitamin A
- Vitamin B$_6$
- Vitamin C
- Vitamin E
- Magnesium
- Selenium
- Zinc
- Coenzyme Q$_{10}$
- Reduced L-glutathione
- DHEA (Dehydroepiandrosterone)

The ten nutrients listed above can help you live a long life without cancer, arthritis or other degenerative diseases. Expect to be full of energy and vigor to live out your dreams without the threat of illness. All you have to do is follow the steps outlined in this chapter.

ZINC: THE THYMUS BOOSTER

The thymus gland is like the orchestra conductor or commanding officer of a very large army. Without a healthy thymus, the immune system can't do the job it's designed to do. Enough T-cells will not mature to go out and fight invaders. Zinc is the most important mineral to the thymus gland. It is so important, in fact, that even if you have a small or malfunctioning thymus, zinc supplements can reverse and rejuvenate it.

Causes of Zinc Deficiency

- vegetarian diets (phytates in plant foods inhibit zinc)
- low red meat consumption
- low consumption of seafood
- dieting, especially high-carbohydrate diets
- copper toxicity
- low stomach acid
- digestive disorders
- aging

In an article in *Nutrition Reviews*, Ananda Prasad states that there are more than 300 enzyme systems in the body that require zinc. A deficiency can result in poor growth as seen in children, small testes, anorexia, slow wound healing, delayed puberty and skin problems. Especially important to the scope of this book is the impact that zinc deficiency has on the immune system. Zinc is required for cell-mediated immunity and proper cell division as well as for DNA synthesis. Prasad also found that when 30 mg of zinc was provided daily to zinc-deficient elderly subjects, levels of interleukin-2 and thymulin increased. Remember, interleukin-2 authorizes cytotoxic T-cells to attack invaders.

Zinc deficiency causes a reduction in T-cells, natural killer cells and thymic hormone. Supplementation with zinc increases the ability of macrophages to digest invaders, dead cells and other debris, and enhances the ability of the immune system to eliminate bacteria. A recent study published in *Nutrition* examined the zinc status of 228 AIDS patients. Low zinc levels were found to be associated with an increased incidence of systemic bacterial infections. It was recommended that patients deficient in zinc take a supplement containing 15 to 60 mg of zinc daily to improve the immune system's antibacterial ability.

Zinc's antiviral activity was examined in a double-blind, placebo-controlled trial with 37 cold-infected subjects. Zinc lozenges containing 23 mg of zinc were taken at two-hour intervals. After seven days, over 85 percent of the participants were symptom free, compared to half of the placebo group. Zinc lozenges are now commonly prescribed for the cold virus, but remember, even too much of a good thing can be bad. One study of 11 subjects who ingested 300 mg (150 mg twice a day) of zinc daily for six weeks found that the immune function was suppressed.

Food sources for zinc include oysters, red meat, shellfish, pumpkinseeds, gingerroot, pecans, Brazil nuts, whole grains, almonds, walnuts, hazelnuts, legumes, garlic, beans and potatoes.

SELENIUM

Without adequate quantities of selenium we are highly susceptible to cancer, viruses and free radical damage. Selenium is one of the most potent free radical scavengers that we call antioxidants. Areas of the world that have low selenium levels have correspondingly high levels of cancer and viruses. For example, Professor Harold Foster of the University of Victoria, British Columbia, found that breast cancer rates were strongly correlated to soil selenium levels. As well, Zaire, Africa, which has extremely low soil selenium levels, has unusually high rates of HIV infection. Also interesting is a study published in the *Journal of the American College of Nutrition* that showed dormant coxsackievirus B_3 become active and virulent in selenium-deficient mice. The researchers noted that the public health implications of this are significant with the increase in RNA viruses such as AIDS, polio and influenza. (Retrovirus is a virus that contains RNA as its genetic information, but uses double-strand DNA as an intermediate in its replication. Certain retrovirus can cause tumors in infected cells.) Optimal selenium levels may have profound protective effects against the activation of viruses.

Selenium is essential to the production of a powerful enzyme called glutathione peroxidase, which is important in detoxifying the body of environmental toxins. Selenium deficiency causes poor resistance to viruses and bacteria, and reduces T-cell activity and antibody production. Imagine an immune system that is unable to mobilize its T-cells and natural killer cells to destroy pathogenic bacteria and viruses. This is exactly what occurs in a selenium-deficient immune system.

Selenium's importance in the production of the enzyme glutathione peroxidase was examined in a 1997 research study on HIV-infected individuals. It was found that the HIV virus replicates more rapidly in a cell that is deficient in this important enzyme. Selenium supplementation was also found to increase IL-2, which is important in activating natural killer cell activity. This nutrient is important in conditions such as HIV and autoimmune disorders to keep the immune system in balance. An overactivation of self-damaging cytokines and free radicals may be kept in check with selenium supplementation.

Another study involving rheumatoid arthritis patients showed that selenium supplementation is important in reducing the production of inflammatory prostaglandins and leukotrienes, as well as free radicals, factors which are thought to cause most of the damage seen in rheumatoid arthritis.

Brazil nuts, still in the shell, are an excellent food source of selenium. One or two Brazil nuts daily provide adequate selenium to the diet. Brazil nuts are also rich in phytosterols, another important nutrient for the immune system. Selenium should be supplemented in doses of 100 mcg to 200 mcg daily to enhance immune function.

VITAMIN E

Vitamin E, in conjunction with selenium and vitamin C, is the most potent immune protector. It increases resistance to infection, cell-mediated immunity and phagocytosis (the ability of cells to digest), and reduces damage caused by stress. Known as the fountain of youth, this vitamin is an active antioxidant with so many protective benefits that we should never forget to take a food supplement containing 400 IU (International Units) daily. Not only does vitamin E boost the immune system, it also has a significant benefit in cardiovascular disease, diabetes, cancer, skin disorders, arthritis, premenstrual syndrome (PMS), menopausal symptoms, inflammation, and the list goes on.

An increase in T-cells, interleukin-2 and tumor necrosis factor (TNF) and a reduction in inflammatory prostaglandins, all important immune factors, was found in a study of ten subjects taking 1,000 mg of vitamin C and 400 mg of vitamin E for 28 days. The synergistic effect of vitamin E and vitamin C is of special importance as vitamin C transforms oxidized vitamin E, making its benefits available. Combined, vitamins C and E offer a formidable defense against immune-damaging factors.

Low or deficient levels of vitamin E in the body are related to certain cancers, especially those of the gastrointestinal tract and lungs. Vitamin E appears to prevent cancers of the breast and prostate by inhibiting cancer cells from multiplying. A 14-year study involving 5,000 British women showed that low blood levels of vitamin E increased breast cancer risk by 500 percent. Vitamin E's free radical scavenging abilities can reduce the risk of cancer by 50 percent with a daily dosage of 400 IU. Large-scale studies now provide evidence that vitamin E supplementation can lower the risk of colon cancer.

Another study found that when elderly people living on their own were given 200 mg of vitamin E for 235 days, their B-cell activity increased. A sixfold increase in antibodies to the hepatitis B virus was found when compared to the placebo group. They also found that the 200-mg daily dose increased antibodies to both tetanus and pneumonia vaccines.

Vitamin E is difficult to obtain in therapeutic quantities from the foods we eat due to grain-milling and food-processing methods. You would need to consume 9 pounds of almonds to get enough vitamin E to boost immunity. Take a vitamin E supplement to ensure you are adequately protected. Choose a supplement that provides vitamin E in the natural d-alpha tocopherol with mixed tocopherols, preferably with a high gamma tocopherol content.

VITAMIN C

The late Linus Pauling spent half his life extolling the benefits of vitamin C. Pauling died at the age of 93 due to prostate cancer, but maintained that his life was extended by several decades due to his consumption of vitamin C. He is not alone in this belief. Emanuel Cheraskin, MD, DMD, Abram Hoffer, MD, PhD and others have also focused their attention on this life-enhancing nutrient. Indeed, no other vitamin has received as much attention as vitamin C. Thousands of research papers and almost as many books have been written about this essential nutrient. Emanuel Cheraskin titled his book *Vitamin C: Who Needs It?*, and then provided more than 50 double-blind studies (see page 120 for explanation of double-blind studies) to prove that we all need vitamin C. In one of these studies, Prinz and associates from the University of Witwatersrand Medical School, South Africa, gave 25 medical students a gram of Vitamin C as ascorbic acid daily for 75 days. An increase in the antibodies IgA and IgM was noted in the group given ascorbic acid, and no immune-enhancing effect was shown in the group that received no vitamin C.

Vitamin C Facts

- The National Institutes of Health, Bethesda, Maryland, state that only 9 percent of Americans are in an optimal vitamin C state.

- One cigarette smoked eliminates 25 mg of vitamin C from the body.

- 10-gram doses of vitamin C daily may make birth control pills ineffective.

- 1,000 mg of vitamin C per day increases sperm motility and fertility.

- In order to get the minimum requirement of vitamin C, you would have to eat five vine-ripened fruits and vegetables.

As early as 1949, Frederick Klenner published a paper in *Southern Medicine and Surgery* on the effectiveness of vitamin C on polio and other viruses. He was curing—yes, *curing*—polio when nothing else worked. Klenner gave patients ascorbic acid intravenously in high doses and unrelentingly until the virus was eradicated. At the time this information was published, the Salk vaccine had just been introduced. Klenner believed that polio was not as dangerous as it appeared to be and that marshaling the body's natural immunity would have been a safer route than vaccination.

Vitamin C provides protection against viral infection by strengthening connective tissue and neutralizing toxic substances that are released by phagocytes. Its direct antiviral action appears to be through the suppression of virus replication and the annihilation of virus-infected cells. Research confirms that vitamin C is antiviral, antibacterial and anticancer. It is known that PGE1, a prostaglandin that plays a major role in regulating T-cell function, is enhanced by vitamin C. Vitamin C enhances one of the complement enzymes, C_1 esterase, without which the entire enzymatic cascade of complement would not occur and non-self cells would not be destroyed. Tests show that taking as little as 1,200 mg of vitamin C per day increased T-cell activity, and 500 mg per day increased glutathione levels by 50 percent. As mentioned earlier, glutathione is extremely important to immune function by eliminating toxic substances from the body, enhancing cellular oxygen and activating enzymatic reactions.

One study evaluated 55 patients who had toxic chemical exposure. Initial evaluations determined low to inadequate natural killer cell and B-cell activity. Each patient was given 60 mg per kilogram body weight of vitamin C . Immune parameters were measured every 24 hours. In 78 percent of patients, natural killer cell activity increased tenfold and B-cell function improved to normal after only 24 hours of supplementation with vitamin C. Researchers believed that vitamin C would be effective in treating malignant tumors and in preventing or delaying infections.

Foods high in vitamin C include brussels sprouts, cabbage, cauliflower, collard greens, mustard greens, broccoli, black currants, kale, parsley, chili peppers, sweet red and green peppers.

Vitamin C to Bowel Tolerance

How much is too much vitamin C? Robert Cathcart, MD, states that each individual has his or her own ascorbate limit, which is determined by stress, nutritional status and current state of health. To determine your personal ascorbate requirements, start taking gram doses of vitamin C until your bowels become loose, then cut back until your bowel movements are normal. This is your personal ascorbate requirement. Depending on your current health and lifestyle choices, this level may fluctuate from day to day or week to week. The Recommended Daily Allowance (RDA) of vitamin C is 60 mg per day. Most individuals require much more.

VITAMIN A

Vitamin A is a clear immune booster. If you are deficient in this vitamin, you will be prone to infections, especially colds and flus. Wounds will not heal as quickly, including stomach ulcers. Vitamin A has two very important functions relating to the immune system: it normalizes cell division and helps mucus membranes maintain their structural integrity to keep invaders out.

Vitamin A deficiency causes the thymus to shrink, resulting in an impaired immune system. With inadequate quantities of vitamin A in the body, antibody production will be reduced and T-cells will not be able to fight invaders. So important is this nutrient to our immune system that deficiencies have been associated with higher death rates in those with infections. One study involving

AIDS patients found that when vitamin A blood levels were low, helper T-cell levels were also low. With supplementation of vitamin A, helper T-cells increased along with a subsequent improvement in immune function.

Many cancer studies show that pharmacological (above standard recommended) doses of vitamin A used in cancer therapies alleviate the immunosuppressive effects of chemotherapy and radiation therapy, thereby allowing the patient's immune system to help fight the cancer.

One caveat of vitamin A use is, in high doses of more than 50,000 IU daily over many years, toxicity can occur. Beta-carotene, a precursor to vitamin A, is a safer nutrient to be taken on a daily basis. (See chapter 4 for discussion of carotenoids.)

Foods high in vitamin A include dark green, orange and red fruits and vegetables.

COENZYME Q_{10}: THE SPARK OF LIFE

Important to energy production in the body, coenzyme Q_{10} is often referred to as the spark of life. By the time we are 50 years old, our CoQ_{10} level is half what it was when we were 20. Scientists believe that low levels of coenzyme Q_{10} are directly related to an increase in heart damage, since the heart muscle is rich in CoQ_{10}.

This powerful antioxidant in doses of 30 to 60 mg has an immune-enhancing effect by increasing antibody production. It has also been found to minimize the effects of chemotherapy-induced toxicity. Research shows that macrophage activity is increased with CoQ_{10} supplementation, and that CoQ_{10} has antiviral, antibacterial and antitumor effects.

In a study published in *Clinical Investigator*, Dr. K. Folkers found that the antibody IgG was dramatically increased with a daily dose of only 60 mg of CoQ_{10}. So dramatic was the increase, Folkers felt that age-associated decline in immune function could be easily reversed with CoQ_{10}.

Lockwood and fellow researchers found that CoQ_{10} in doses over 300 mg per day inhibited tumor growth in breast cancer, with several patients experiencing complete tumor regression. Although the mechanism of action was not determined, the results are promising enough to encourage all women to supplement their diets with adequate levels of CoQ_{10} as a breast cancer protective nutrient.

CoQ_{10} should be supplemented in capsule form as it is difficult to obtain an immune-enhancing level from the food we eat. Fatty fish such as sardines, organ meats and peanuts contain CoQ_{10}, but you would have to consume pounds of these foods to obtain adequate levels of the nutrient. Thirty milligrams of CoQ_{10} per day is the maintenance dose, but over 320 mg have been used to treat breast cancer without side effects. (See chapter 11 for a further discussion.)

GLUTATHIONE: THE FREE RADICAL FIGHTER

No other antioxidant is as important to overall health as glutathione. It is the regenerator of immune cells and the most valuable detoxifying agent in the body. Low levels are associated with early aging and even death. Optimal levels make your immune cells extremely efficient. Glutathione is composed of three amino acids—cysteine, glutamic acid and glycine. It is produced in every cell with the aid of selenium, magnesium and vitamin C, and is abundantly found in foods.

Free radical damage goes unchecked without adequate cell levels of glutathione. Imagine a stampede of cattle damaging everything in their path. This is what occurs in the body of someone even moderately deficient in glutathione. One study found that when elderly patients with mild glutathione deficiencies were given 75 mg daily, their T-cell activity increased dramatically, they felt healthier and had more energy. Another study found that higher glutathione levels were associated with fewer illnesses, lower cholesterol, lower blood pressure and a greater feeling of well-being.

A review article published in the *Annals of Pharmacology* stated that glutathione is important in DNA synthesis and repair, protein and prostaglandin synthesis, amino acid transport, detoxification of toxins and carcinogens, enhancement of the immune system and protection from oxidation and enzyme activations. People who suffer from environmental allergies, especially acute chemical sensitivities, can alleviate allergic reactions quickly with supplementation of reduced L-glutathione in a daily dose of 200 to 500 mg.

Oxidative stress may be one reason for HIV disease progression, by causing the virus to reproduce, increasing immune inflammatory responses, increasing cell death, increasing toxicity and chronic weight loss. Due to its powerful antioxidant properties, glutathione reduces oxidative stress. In test tube studies, glutathione killed the AIDS virus. Unfortunately, in humans, this does not occur, but it does have important immune-enhancing effects for those afflicted with the virus.

Glutathione Benefits—the Nutrient of Youth

- keeps cholesterol from oxidizing
- eliminates carcinogens
- improves T-cell function
- controls insulin
- halts inflammatory responses
- reduces allergic reactions
- revs up the immune system
- protects against cancer
- detoxifies alcohol

To ensure adequate blood levels of glutathione, use 75 mg of the most active form, reduced L-glutathione (99 percent of glutathione in human tissue is in the reduced active state). Include the cofactors selenium, magnesium and vitamin C. Many individuals believe that glutathione cannot be absorbed intact via the gut but several valuable studies now show that not only is it absorbed but it is important for its antioxidant activity in the gastrointestinal tract both in and outside of cells. Glutathione's powerful detoxifying action can also protect us against ultraviolet radiation, X rays, peroxides and the toxic effects of alcohol and prescription medications. Antioxidants are the key to anti-aging, immune enhancement and the control of scavenging free radicals.

Food sources of glutathione include the cruciferous vegetables brussels sprouts, cabbage, cauliflower, and broccoli. These vegetables are rich in phytonutrients that also boast potent antioxidant properties. Watermelon and avocado are the richest food sources of glutathione.

VITAMIN B$_6$

Required for maintaining hormone levels, a healthy immune and nervous system, prostaglandin formation and the formation of proteins, vitamin B$_6$ is essential to health. Moderate vitamin B$_6$ deficiency is so common that everyone needs to supplement their diet with the nutrient. More than 50 enzymatic reactions depend on vitamin B$_6$.

Immune enhancement relies upon adequate vitamin B_6. Without enough the thymus will shrink and a reduction in the amount of thymulin will result. T-cell activity will diminish along with B-cells and antibodies. Interleukin-2 is also reduced, disabling natural killer cells, which raises the risk of infection and cancer, and compromises the immune system. Vitamin B_6 deficiency essentially cripples the army of the immune system. It is like an army without weapons waiting for attackers to descend.

One study of HIV-infected patients found that low vitamin B_6 was associated with a decrease in immune function. When relatively low doses of the vitamin were added, immune function increased tenfold.

Vitamin B_6 should be taken in conjunction with the other B vitamins in a complex. This is the way they are found in nature and each has a synergistic effect on the other. Pyridoxal-5-phosphate, the active form of vitamin B_6, is already broken down to its reduced state, making it bio-available. Those with liver problems or lacking the enzyme to break down vitamin B_6 should use this form of the vitamin. Magnesium is a cofactor required for vitamin B_6 absorption. If you use a nutritional supplement of B_6, look for one with added magnesium. To maintain immunity, 50 mg of vitamin B_6 is required.

Food sources of B vitamins are meat, fish and poultry, grains, nuts and seeds, soybeans, green leafy vegetables and potatoes.

MAGNESIUM

Although magnesium is not a clear immune-enhancing nutrient, it is included in this discussion because it is responsible for more than 300 enzymatic reactions in the body. Deficiencies are common and result in heart attacks, kidney stones, cancer, premenstrual syndrome (PMS) and insomnia. Supplementation lowers blood pressure, prevents diabetes, keeps bones strong and extends life.

A recent report in the *American Journal of Clinical Pathology* found that magnesium deficiency causes an increase in pro-inflammatory conditions and an excess production of free radicals seen in chronic fatigue syndrome, fibromyalgia and rheumatoid conditions. Free radical damage, as discussed earlier, is the main factor in cellular destruction of body tissues. Magnesium-deficient cells release more pro-inflammatory cytokines, which then cause more free radical production and further damage, as is seen in rheumatoid arthritis.

Many physicians recommend a dose of 6 mg of magnesium per kilogram of body weight. An average daily dose is 350 mg. If you drink caffeinated beverages or are under stress, you will require a higher dose. Calcium and potassium should also be supplemented along with magnesium as these nutrients work synergistically.

Food sources of magnesium are tofu, legumes, seeds and nuts, green leafy vegetables and whole unrefined grains. Diets high in dairy products and meat are low in magnesium.

DHEA—THE IMMUNE HORMONE

Over the last decade, DHEA, dehydroepiandrosterone, has enjoyed widespread popularity as an antiaging nutrient. Along with its ability to control age-related disorders, it helps to repair and maintain tissues, control allergic reactions and symptoms, and most important, balance the activity of the immune system.

This super hormone is secreted by the adrenal glands, then converted into several other hormones required by the body—testosterone, dihydro-testosterone, androstenedione, estradiol and estrone. Its ability to convert into so many other hormones has given DHEA the distinction of being a "mother hormone."

The body makes DHEA from cholesterol and betasitosterol, which it then turns into pregnenolone and 17 alpha hydroxy pregnenolone before it

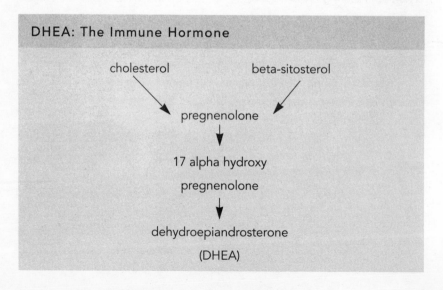

DHEA: The Immune Hormone

cholesterol   beta-sitosterol

pregnenolone

17 alpha hydroxy
pregnenolone

dehydroepiandrosterone
(DHEA)

becomes DHEA. As we age, this conversion often becomes impaired. Our levels of DHEA and the corresponding male and female sex hormones decline. By the time we reach our fifties, our DHEA levels are half what they were when we were 20. Sexual dysfunction, muscle shrinkage, memory loss, degenerative diseases and poor immune function are only some of the problems that scientists feel are associated with the loss of this potent hormone.

DHEA and Diabetes

Insulin sensitivity declines as we age, allowing glucose to remain in the blood. High levels of glucose in the blood cause significant side effects including neuropathy (nerve damage) and atherosclerosis (hardening of the arteries). Studies involving insulin-dependent diabetics (Type I diabetes) found that DHEA levels are very low in those afflicted. When supplemental DHEA in a dose of 50 mg was added, hardening of the arteries was reduced and insulin sensitivity increased.

DHEA and Immune Function

One study involving postmenopausal women and immune function found that when DHEA was added, there was a corresponding increase in the level of all immune cells. Researchers believe that this action may account for DHEA's anticancer properties in non-estrogen-dominant cancers.

Another interesting study looked at DHEA levels in elderly subjects and the effects of the flu vaccine post–DHEA supplementation. Ironically, the flu vaccine given to aging people to protect them against the flu does not work because the person's aging immune system is unable to make antibodies against the vaccine. When the over 65-year-old volunteers were given DHEA along with their flu shot, the immune response significantly improved.

We know that DHEA is integrally linked to immune function. When DHEA levels are low, cortisol, the stress hormone, is often found to be high. DHEA seems to be a protective factor against the negative effects of cortisol. High cortisol levels increase the release of interleukin-6, promoting inflammation and destruction of body tissues. DHEA is important in keeping cortisol in balance.

DHEA and Lupus

In one study, female volunteers with systemic lupus erythematosus (SLE) were given 200 mg of DHEA for up to six months. All the women in the study noted overall improvement in the way they felt and the SLE Disease Activity Index score (a way of rating severity and presence of the disease) was improved significantly. Lupus is a serious autoimmune disorder (see chapter 9) with few effective treatments. DHEA offered relief of many symptoms associated with the disease with only one noted side effect, mild skin inflammation.

DHEA and AIDS

For information on DHEA and HIV/AIDS, see chapter 11.

Dosage

DHEA is available in several forms: capsules, liquids and sprays. For those over 60 years of age we recommend you begin with a low dose of 5 mg and increase gradually only to achieve the desired effect. For those who live in Canada and cannot purchase DHEA due to government restrictions in the sale of the product, Sterinol is a precursor to pregnenolone, which is then converted into DHEA. One capsule 3 times daily is recommended.

DHEA can have side effects if taken in high doses; these include acne, oily skin, facial hair growth in women, deepening of the voice and mood swings. All side effects reverse to normal when DHEA supplementation is discontinued or reduced to appropriate levels. Men who have prostate cancer or women with estrogen-dominant cancers should avoid supplementation with DHEA. Sterinol does not cause the above side effects as the body will only convert the amount of DHEA that it needs.

Daily Dosages of the Ten Immune-Boosting Nutrients	
NUTRIENT	DOSAGE
Vitamin C	1,000 mg or to bowel tolerance
Vitamin A	5,000 IU
Vitamin E	400–800 IU
Zinc	15 mg
Selenium	100 mcg
Coenzyme Q_{10}	60 mg
Reduced L-glutathione	75 mg–150 mg
Vitamin B_6 (in a B complex)	50 mg
Magnesium	100 mg
DHEA	5 mg increased until symptoms abate

Vitamin and mineral supplements alone cannot provide you with all the immune-boosting benefits you require to fight off cancer, viruses, parasites and bacteria as well as keep you fit and youthful. Good nutrition is the foundation for longevity and strong immunity. The next two chapters will provide you with the nutrition facts you need to optimize immunity, prevent disease and live a long life.

PHYTONUTRIENTS: POWERFUL IMMUNE SYSTEM PROTECTION

Phytonutrients have the ability to halt a cell from converting to a cancerous cell.

—American Institute for Cancer Research

Your mother knew what she was talking about when she told you to eat your fruits and vegetables. Fresh, organic fruits, vegetables, seeds and nuts not only provide high fiber, vitamins and minerals but are rich in powerful disease-fighting substances called phytonutrients. These biologically active substances give plants their color, flavor and natural resistance to disease. The most significant benefit to human health is the ability of phytonutrients to boost immunity, slow the aging process and combat disease, especially cancer.

The word "phytochemical" is often used interchangeably with the term "phytonutrient"; it comes from the Greek *phyto*, meaning plant. Currently, beta-carotene is the most researched phytonutrient, with phytosterols following a close second. Indeed, researchers are discovering new phytonutrients almost daily. The following plant nutrients are the most well known: phytosterols, including beta-sitosterol and beta-sitosterolin; carotenoids, including lycopene; phytoestrogens, especially genistein and daidzein; indoles and lignans; flavonoids, including quercetin, silymarin and anthocyanidins.

To ensure adequate protection from disease, we must eat 7 to 10 half-cup servings of fresh, organic fruits, vegetables, seeds and nuts daily. Food processing destroys phytonutrients, especially in seed and nut oils. While cooking does not destroy these nutrients, they are reduced; and when we throw away the cooking water, we are often throwing out the most important substances. Freezing food releases certain enzymes, destroying the health-promoting substances. What this means is fresh is definitely best.

Supercharging the immune system is of paramount importance to live a vibrant, healthy life. Eating the required amounts of fruits and vegetables is the first step to disease protection. For people who just can't seem to consume the fruits and vegetables they need, supplementation is essential. Fortunately, food supplements are available that provide most of the above phytochemicals either singly or in combination.

FLAVONOIDS

Next to carotenoids, flavonoids are the most prevalent phytonutrient in the plant kingdom. Discovered by Albert Szent-Gyorgi in 1936, they include quercetin, Pycnogenol™, catechin, rutin, anthocyanidin, luteolin, kampferol, astragelin and hesperidin.

Flavonoids are potent antioxidants that prevent the formation of free radicals. Flavonoids also prevent inflammatory leukotrienes from causing joint pain and destruction. Many flavonoids are more effective than vitamins C and E. Flavonoids also improve the absorbability of vitamin C, which is the reason they are often combined in nutritional supplements that contain vitamin C.

Flavonoids stop the action of the enzyme hyaluronidase; this enzyme is responsible for degrading connective tissue ground substances, which allows pathogens and bacteria into the cell. Think of this ground substance as a rubber balloon; as long as the exterior of the balloon is intact, it will hold air or water, but the moment it is compromised, the interior is open to the outside. The anti-hyaluronidase action of the flavonoids catechin, rutin, quercetin and hesperidin helps defend connective tissue and thereby strengthen the immune system, halt inflammation and ward off bacteria.

Flavonoids are especially beneficial in treating diabetics, as these phytonutrients have the ability to lower blood sugar levels. They also slow the release of histamine in allergic responses, especially in cases of anaphylactic shock. Flavonoids in doses of 500 mg, three times daily, are known to calm asthmatic and allergic conditions.

Most important to the health of the immune system, flavonoids stimulate T-cell formation and lymphocyte transformation. It is also thought that flavonoids inhibit a substance known as P-450 aromatase, which causes regression of estrogen-sensitive tumors, especially breast tumors. Other cancer enzyme receptors are also inactivated or halted by the addition of flavonoids to the daily diet.

Liver-damaging endotoxins caused by bacteria that are not dealt with by the immune system are also eliminated by the activity of flavonoids. Antibacterial and antiviral properties are well documented, but the newest and most exciting research focuses on the protection that flavonoids offer to capillaries. These special phytochemicals are now being used to treat vision problems including night blindness, and to strengthen and repair broken capillaries, varicose veins and cardiac irregularities arising from a decrease in blood flow and arterial blockages.

Foods containing flavonoids should be eaten daily. Flavonoid-rich foods include broccoli, grapes, carrots, onions, peppers, green tea, tangerines, elderberries, blueberries, bilberries, apples, all citrus fruits and Gingko biloba.

CAROTENOIDS

Currently more than 600 different carotenoids have been identified. The most abundant and well known are lutein, canthaxanthin, zeaxanthin, alpha-carotene, lycopene and cryptoxanthin. Dark green, yellow, red and orange vegetables and fruits are rich in carotenoids. Most carotenoids have no or low vitamin A activity but offer superior antioxidant activity that protects the body against cataracts, macular degeneration and skin damage. They also have powerful anticancer properties, reducing the risk for breast, prostate, cervix and colon cancer. Moreover, carotenoids destroy and neutralize free radicals before they have a chance to damage cells, thereby staving off cardiovascular disease and diabetes.

The following lists natural sources of carotenoids.

- Beta-carotene: apricots, carrots, peaches, sweet potatoes
- Alpha-carotene: carrots, pumpkins, red and yellow peppers, yellow corn
- Cryptoxanthin: papayas, peaches, tangerines, oranges
- Lutein: kale, collard greens, spinach, broccoli, mustard greens
- Zeaxanthin: cress leaf, Swiss chard, chicory leaf, beet greens, okra
- Lycopene: tomatoes, watermelon, guava

Lycopene: the New Kid on the Block

Lycopene is a powerful antioxidant that halts damage caused by free radicals. Along with lutein and zeaxanthin it slows macular degeneration in the eyes.

A report released by Harvard University states that men can reduce the likelihood of prostate cancer by 22 percent by eating between 4 and 7 tomato-based foods weekly. Another study published in the *Journal of the National Cancer Institute* found that men could reduce the risk of prostate cancer by 35 percent by eating 10 or more servings of lycopene-rich tomato products per week. Sun-ripened tomatoes, watermelon, guava and pink grapefruit are richer in lycopene than those picked green and allowed to ripen during transit, and sun-dried tomatoes are even higher in lycopene content.

Lycopene is a fat-soluble carotenoid. Drizzle a little flaxseed oil or olive oil on top of fresh, sliced tomatoes or add it to your tomato sauce just before serving to ensure you absorb more lycopene.

Immune-Boosting Beta-Carotene

The most researched carotenoid is beta-carotene, also known as provitamin A. Beta-carotene is converted into vitamin A by the body, but unlike vitamin A, beta-carotene is not toxic. If too many carotenoids are consumed, a yellowing of the skin occurs. This discoloration quickly disappears when carotenoid consumption is reduced. Babies who eat a lot of carrots and dark vegetables often get this discoloration on the soles of the feet, palms of the hands and the tip of the nose. It is nothing to be concerned about and will fade and disappear as soon as the carotenoid-rich foods are reduced.

Beta-carotene is the carotenoid responsible for the orange or red color of fruits and vegetables. Foods rich in beta-carotene include apricots, carrots, yams, sweet potatoes, squash, peaches and mangoes. Include plenty of carotene-rich foods in your daily diet as they are known to reduce the risk of developing cancers of the colon, esophagus, pancreas, stomach and throat. They also boost the immune system, and enhance the response of T-cells and B-cells. A study published in the *Journal of Nutrition* found that the number of natural killer cells and B-cells (antibody cells) were improved in HIV patients supplemented with a low dose of 60 mg of beta-carotene daily for four months.

In most cases, foods are your best source of phytonutrients. In the case of carotenoids, however, the jury is still out on whether we absorb or convert to vitamin A enough carotenoids to provide a protective effect. Until we are sure, or if you are not eating enough fruits and vegetables, supplement with a carotenoid product that is derived from *Dunaliella salina algae* (Betatene®) grown in Australia. It contains at least 5 percent of the mixed carotenoids mentioned above. Also look for carotenoid supplements that contain lycopene as well. You can purchase this type of supplement from your health food store. It is distributed by Twin Labs, Klaire Laboratories, Jarrow Formulas, Solgar and Carlson. (See Appendix I)

PHYTOSTEROLS

Phytosterols are plant sterols that include beta-sitosterol and its glucoside beta-sitosterolin, as well as campesterol, brassicasterol, stigmasterol, ergosterol and avenasterol. Among the various sterols, B-sitosterol, campesterol and stigmasterol have the greatest nutritional importance. They make up 45 to 90 percent of the total sterols of edible plants. Beta-sitosterol and beta-sitosterolins (sterols and sterolins) were identified and isolated as early as 1922. Since then, hundreds of research papers have been published on the health benefits of these substances.

Sterols are plant fats very similar in structure to the animal fat cholesterol except they have an extra ethyl group on the side chain. All plants, including fruits, vegetables, seeds and nuts, contain sterols and sterolins. These sterols never exist on their own in nature; they are always found in combination with their glucoside, which is called beta-sitosterolin (sterolin). This glucoside has a synergistic effect along with the sterol and plays an important role in immune-modulating activity. Without the glucoside, the sterols are not effective in treating disease and boosting the immune system. Sterinol combines both types of sterols in the correct ratio for optimal activity.

STEROLS: POWERFUL IMMUNE ENHANCERS

Sterols are absorbed from the gastrointestinal tract with less efficiency than cholesterol, and may actually interfere with the normal absorption of dietary and/or biliary cholesterol. Due to this effect, plant sterols, especially B-sitosterol, in high doses, are being used as a treatment for high cholesterol (hypercholesterolaemia) to compete with the normal absorption of cholesterol.

The unique combination of sterols and sterolins called Sterinol have also been studied for the treatment of benign prostatic hypertrophy (BPH), HIV, tuberculosis, and for the treatment of exercise-induced stress, as seen in marathon runners. New research is under way to confirm the effects seen in individual patient cases for rheumatoid arthritis, rhinitis and sinusitis, chronic fatigue syndrome, HIV, asthma, cervical cancer and hepatitis C. Preliminary results verify what has been described in many of the case histories throughout this book. Look for exciting research to be released late 1999.

Rheumatoid arthritis, one of the most debilitating and difficult-to-treat diseases of our day, has finally met its match with Sterinol. In recent studies, Sterinol was found to inhibit the secretion of inflammatory cytokines, which resulted in a decrease of the production and release of both IL-6 and TNF-alpha, two factors responsible for inflammation in rheumatoid arthritis. The disorders mentioned above are discussed in subsequent chapters, and the importance of plant sterols in the functioning of the immune system will become very clear.

Foods Rich in Sterols and Sterolins

Raw unprocessed nuts and seeds and their oils are the richest natural sources of sterols and sterolins. Standard oil processing methods destroy the sterols and sterolins contained in the foods, stripping the finished product of any health-giving properties. Food processing, including freezing fruits and vegetables, destroys the glucoside molecules (Sterolins) attached to the sterols, which eliminates the immune-enhancing factor.

Boiling vegetables causes the sterols and sterolins to be released into the cooking water, which is then discarded. Moreover, diets consumed in industrialized countries are deficient in fruits and vegetables and therefore lack the benefits provided by nature's powerful phytochemicals. Choose the foods that are the richest in sterols from the following chart and make sure you incorporate them into your diet every day. Less than 5 percent of the sterols and sterolins are absorbed from food sources. For insurance that you are getting your daily dose of protective sterols and sterolins, take three capsules of Sterinol daily.

Sterol Content of Common Foods

Food	beta-sitosterol & beta-sitosterolin (mg/100 g edible portion)	campesterol	stigmasterol
Vegetables			
Asparagus	14	3	5
Barley	98	33	101
Beetroot	13	0	6
Brussels sprouts	17	6	1
Cabbage	7	2	2
Carrots	7	1	3
Cauliflower	12	3	2
Cucumbers	14	0	0
Gingerroot	10	1	4
Squash, white	89	2	0
Lettuce, romaine	21	2	11
Melons	16	0	0
Okra	15	3	6
Onions	15	12	1
Peas	108	0	0
Peppers, red	7	3	2
Potatoes, sweet	8	3	1
Potatoes, white	40	0	0
Pumpkin	12	0	0
Radish greens	22	6	0
Soybeans	30	9	11
Taro	11	3	6
Turnip greens	9	2	0
Yams	7	2	2

Food	beta-sitosterol & beta-sitosterolin (mg/100 g edible portion)	campesterol	stigmasterol
Fruits			
Apples	11	1	0
Apricots	16	1	0
Bananas	11	2	3
Cherries	12	0	0
Figs	27	1	2
Grapefruit	13	2	2
Lemons	8	0	0
Oranges, navel	17	4	2
Peaches	6	1	1
Pears	7	0	0
Pomegranates	16	trace	trace
Strawberries	10	trace	trace
Seeds and Nuts			
Almonds	122	5	3
Cashews	130	13	tr
Chestnuts	18	2	2
Coconuts, meat	27	3	7
Pecans	88	4	2
Pine nuts	84	14	trace
Pistachios	90	6	2
Sesame seeds	443	91	78
Sunflower seeds	349	61	75
Walnuts	87	6	0
Vegetable Oils			
Cocoa butter	59	26	9

Food	beta-sitosterol & beta-sitosterolin (mg/100 g edible portion)	campesterol	stigmasterol
Flaxseed	46	9	29
Olive (France)	91	1	3
Olive (Italy)	84	1	3
Safflower	52	9	13
Soybean	53	20	20
Sunflower	60	8	8
Wheat germ	67	trace	22
Legumes and Beans			
Azuki	37	1	36
Broad	95	8	9
Kidney	91	3	31
Mung	13	2	8
Peanuts	142	24	23
Grains			
Buckwheat	164	20	8
Corn	120	32	21
Rice bran	735	257	289
Whole wheat	40	27	0
Spices, dry			
Clove	242	0	14
Fenugreek	100	18	7
Ginger	56	10	18
Oregano	177	12	15
Paprika	119	29	18
Thyme	152	3	8

Food	beta-sitosterol & beta-sitosterolin (mg/100 g edible portion)	campesterol	stigmasterol
Fish and Seafood	Total sterols		
Haddock	97		
Pollock	80		
Salmon	99		
Shrimp	209		
Lobster	171		
Crab	244		
Oyster	362		
Clams	518		
Scallops	681		

In order to consume 60 mg of plant sterols per day, you would have to eat about 500 to 700 g of fresh fruits and vegetables, 200 g of whole wheat flour without additives, or 250 g of potatoes (not boiled). To achieve maximum immunity, you would have to double this daily requirement.

In his article "The Importance of Sitosterol and Sitosterolin in Human and Animal Nutrition," published in the South African Journal of Science, Karl Pegel (see chapter 1) states that plant sterols are found either singly or in combination in such popular herbal remedies as Serenoa repens and Pygeum africanum, Harpagophytum procumbens, commonly known as devil's claw, Silybum marianum, known as milk thistle, Gingko biloba, Panax ginseng, Siberian ginseng and echinacea. Along with the sterols and sterolins, these herbs also contain other important phytonutrients such as ginsenosides, bilobalides, silymarin and echinacosides. Unfortunately, they are not in the correct ratio as needed for an immune-enhancing effect.

PHYTOESTROGENS

New research confirms that the daily consumption of soy products reduces risk of certain cancers, especially breast and prostate cancers. Asian cultures whose diets are rich in soy foods (30 pounds per person per year) have one-third less prostate cancer and one-quarter less breast cancer than North Americans. The American Cancer Society encourages the use of soy products in the diet. Soy products contain isoflavones, daidzen and genistein as well as protease inhibitors, all of which are powerful anticancer phytochemicals.

Genistein and daidzen, commonly known as phytoestrogens, do not increase estrogen levels in the body but fill the receptor sites on cells meant for estrogen. This action reduces the amount of estrogens produced by the body, thus providing a cancer-protective effect. Estrogens, especially estradiol, are thought to be a causative factor in breast cancer, prostate cancer, menopausal symptoms, osteoporosis, PMS, endometriosis and most hormone-related disorders.

In a double-blind, placebo-controlled study completed in 1998, postmenopausal woman were divided into two groups. One-half of the women were given soy protein and the other half were given a placebo. They were monitored for night sweats and hot flashes over a period of 12 weeks. In the group taking the soy protein, symptoms were significantly reduced.

Genistein prevents blood clots by inhibiting thrombin formation and platelet aggregation, which may cause heart attacks. It also restricts the growth of blood vessels, which are the oxygen and nutrition source around tumors. All isoflavones stop the growth of young malignant tumors, thereby allowing the immune system to mop up these small tumors and eliminate them.

Soy products, a good source of protein, not only contain isoflavones but also folic acid, calcium, magnesium, zinc and lignans. Most important, they contain protease inhibitors, which suppress and stop the spread of cancer cells (metastasis). Protease inhibitors interfere with the normal function of enzymes such as trypsin and chymotrypsin, thereby inhibiting the production of cancer (carcinogenesis).

Soybean products, other beans, peas and seeds are good food sources of isoflavones and sterols and sterolins. It is hoped that in the future, soy drink manufacturers will list the content of these phytonutrients on their food labels so that consumers know what they are buying. Genistein and daidzen are also available in capsule form as food supplements.

Lignans, found predominately in flaxseeds and soybeans, as well as in sesame seeds, grains, fruits and vegetables, also inhibit estrogen. Along with isoflavones, lignans are thought to be responsible for the anticancer effect of soybeans and are the reason for the lower rates of cancer in Asian cultures.

Lignans also decrease the incidence and intensity of hot flashes and improve vaginal dryness. (For a further discussion of lignans, see chapter 5.)

INDOLES

Indoles are similar in action to isoflavones as they inactivate estrogen. There are two important indoles: Indole-3-Carbinol (I3C) and dithiolthiones. The cruciferous vegetables broccoli, brussels sprouts, cabbages, cauliflower, turnips and rutabagas all contain indoles. Broccoli also contains another important phytonutrient called sulphoraphane, which is an extremely potent antioxidant. It is now commonly believed that diets which contain plenty of cruciferous vegetables are cancer protective. The best way to eat these

Phytonutrients Daily Dosages

FLAVONOIDS
Pine Bark Extract (Pycnogenol): 50 mg for maintenance
300–500 mg daily to treat allergies

or

Grape Seed Extract: 50 mg for maintenance
300–500 mg daily to treat allergies

or

Quercetin: 200–500 mg daily

or

Green Tea Extract: 3–5 cups of tea daily or a standardized extract for 80 percent polyphenol 300–500 mg daily

CAROTENOIDS
Beta-carotene: 25,000 IU daily

PHYTOSTEROLS
Sterinol, plant sterols and sterolins: 1 capsule 3 times daily on an empty stomach

PHYTOESTROGENS
Genistein and Daidzen: as recommended on the label
Drink 2 glasses of soy milk daily

vegetables is raw or barely steamed. They need to be chewed very well to activate the enzymes present in the vegetable.

Dithiolthiones activate the release of glutathione from cells in the body. As discussed earlier, glutathione is a potent detoxifier and antioxidant. When glutathione is used by the body to eliminate toxins, it must be replaced either from indole-rich foods or from food supplements of reduced L-glutathione. Research confirms that glutathione clears foreign chemicals such as pesticides, herbicides and xenobiotics (chemicals foreign to the body). Contrary to popular belief, cysteine (acetylcysteine) cannot replace glutathione for this detoxifying function. Glutathione also detoxifies heavy metals such as mercury, lead, cadmium and nickel. One of two mechanisms for metabolizing insulin, and thereby influencing blood glucose levels, is glutathione dependent. (See chapter 3 for more information on the immune enhancing effects of glutathione.)

Indole-3-Carbinol induces estrogen 2-hydroxylation, which decreases the estrogens that cause tumor promotion or initiation.

PROTECT YOUR IMMUNE SYSTEM WITH NATURE'S POWERHOUSES

Now that you understand how important the foods you eat are to the health of your immune system, choose at least 7 to 10 servings per day of the most powerful ones mentioned above. Cancer and other degenerative diseases are preventable if we give our body's defense system what it needs to do its daily work. If you cannot feed your body the food it requires, supplement with the phytochemicals we have been discussing. Try to buy organically grown produce and choose fresh over canned or frozen foods. Make soups, salads and freshly pressed juices a part of your daily diet. Sit down for your meals, chew your food well and enjoy what you eat, especially now that you know how potent certain foods are.

The following chapters will show you how the powerful phytonutrients discussed in this chapter are used to heal diseases such as cancer, arthritis, allergies, colds and influenza, and chronic fatigue syndrome.

5

DISEASE PREVENTION: HOW TO OPTIMIZE IMMUNITY WITH NUTRITION

Over 20,000 research articles have consistently shown that enrichment of the diet with the essential nutrients reverses degenerative disease.

—Kirk Hamilton, *Clinical Pearls*

Increasing rates of cancer, heart and degenerative diseases are a barometer of society's overall ability to fight off disease. As our immune function declines, disease increases. Six major factors determine whether our immune system can keep us healthy or whether it will cause us to succumb to disease. Most of them result from our modern, urban way of life. These factors are:

1. antibiotic overuse and misuse
2. pollution and environmental toxins
3. stress and emotional state
4. genetic makeup
5. lifestyle
6. nutritional status

If the immune system is functioning optimally, it can cope with the first five factors as long as it is given the foods it needs to stay primed. Once the body's nutritional status declines, the immune system also falters and cannot cope with the daily onslaught of toxins, stress and the thousands of germs bombarding it. Deficiencies of only one or two nutrients can result in immune suppression, which ultimately leads to cancer and degenerative diseases. In North America, 65 percent of pregnant women, the elderly and teenagers are nutritionally deficient in their daily requirements of vitamins and minerals.

Malnutrition is mistakenly thought to be a problem of developing countries, not of industrialized ones. Yet, even though we eat more food than required, we suffer from serious nutritional deficiencies. Nutrient-poor food is the mainstay of our North American diet. Our demands for foods that can be left on the shelf for months and served immediately are the basis for our health's demise. So devoid of nutrition are processed foods that we must return nutrients to them before they are packaged. Fast foods, fake foods and junk foods are consumed on a daily basis. Soft drinks outsell "real" fruit juice 4 to 1 as the beverage of choice. Fake fats and sweeteners have insidiously found their way into our diets. Hydrogenated fats and oils, with their killer trans-fatty acids, abound in most packaged foods we eat. Even health-giving seeds and nuts are transformed into cancer and heart disease promoters when processed into oils to prolong their shelf-life. To keep our immune system in peak condition, we must first eliminate these disease-causing foods.

Dr. Abram Hoffer, founder of the *Journal of Orthomolecular Medicine* and pioneer in nutritional medicine and its relationship to nutrition and psychiatric disorders, tells his patients that when they shop for groceries they should avoid the centre aisles of the supermarket. This is where all the processed, packaged, fake, fast and junk foods are located. Frequent the outer aisles of the store, where generally you will find fresh fruits and vegetables, dairy products and eggs, fish and poultry. This is sound advice and the basis for the immune system cure diet.

Nutrient-rich foods must be eaten every day to guard against disease. In many cases, diet alone has been proven to prevent disease: heart disease, cancer and diabetes, among others. Indeed, certain cancer cures have used fruits and vegetables as their foundation. Long-term studies have shown that people who adopt vegetarian diets have lower rates of cancer, live longer and have less heart disease. A sound nutritional platform is where any cure should begin; no herb, vitamin, mineral or phytonutrient alone can cure you of disease without it.

We hear people say, "My grandfather, a farmer, smoked cigarettes every day of his life from age 14 until he died at 75, and he never got cancer, so what gives?" Well, grandfather grew up in an era of few environmental toxins. He ate food fresh from the garden rich in phytonutrients. Bread was made at home with freshly ground ingredients, and butter was made from the cream of his cows. Few people owned freezers and most food was canned or stored in a root cellar. Grandfather also did not have to contend with antibiotics or vaccines; if he contracted a disease, he would either have died or survived with enhanced immune function and lifelong antibodies. He also had daily exercise—working on his farm—to keep his heart in good condition and, most likely, his weight down. Grandfather might have lived to 110 if he hadn't smoked.

The point is, times have changed. Our food supply has been abused and we are suffering the consequences. Diseases unheard of in the early part of the 20th century are being diagnosed—fibromyalgia, chronic fatigue syndrome, celiac disease and a host of autoimmune disorders. Diseases of the nineties we call them. What they really are, are diseases of an immune system gone awry.

Most of us would not think that our gut would be a site of battles fought by the immune system, but half of our total immune cells are located in this area, ready to trap and destroy the antigens that are present in our food supply. As discussed in chapter 2, secretory IgA is a common immune deficiency. It is found in the mucosal lining of the gut and it helps to protect against food-borne antigens. When levels are low, food allergies, irritable bowel syndrome, Crohn's disease and inflammatory conditions persist. A breakdown in this protective barrier can also result in parasite, viral and bacterial infections.

THIRTY DAYS TO BOOST IMMUNITY

Our stomachs are full but our nutrient status is poor. We can easily change this; it is something we have control over. Beating or preventing disease is as easy as choosing the correct foods to bolster your immune system. Add the foods we recommend and eliminate as many of the immune-damaging foods that you can, and within one month you will look and feel the difference.

Foods should be eaten in their whole form whenever possible—for example, the whole orange instead of the concentrated juice, the whole seed and not just the oil extracted from the seed. Nature has formed each food to contain many important components, and we are only now beginning to understand the wisdom in consuming foods in their whole form. New phytonutrients are being discovered regularly and we may never fully understand all of the healing properties found in the whole food. Therefore, consuming food as nature intended is the smartest approach.

Dartmouth Medical School researchers found that whole vegetables were better than isolated food supplements in lowering the risk of colon cancer.

Choose organic foods wherever possible. A 1993 study comparing organic to commercial produce found that commercially grown fruits and vegetables were nutrient poor compared to organic produce. Moreover, commercial produce contained higher amounts of heavy metals than organic foods, most likely as a result of the pesticides and commercial fertilizers used to enhance their growth.

THE US ORGANIC ASSOCIATION STATES THAT:

- Children receive up to 35 percent of their entire lifetime dose of cancer-causing pesticides by the age of five.

- Trace amounts of 17 pesticides were found in the top baby foods sold in the United States.

- Farmworkers experience pesticide-related illness: chronic fatigue and muscle weakness.

- Xenoestrogens, harmful estrogens linked to cancer, are found in pesticides.

- Commercially grown produce contains high levels of toxic heavy metals.

- Commercially grown produce is lower in the minerals selenium and potassium.

- 80 percent of all cancers are caused by toxic agents in our environment.

Many millions of years of health wisdom is programmed into our cells. Successful adaptations were passed on and are carried on our genes. Health depends on 50 essential ingredients including air, water, light, oxygen and food. *Essential* means that our bodies cannot live without them. Since the body cannot make these ingredients, they must therefore be obtained from food or nutrients. The components essential to human health that we can obtain from food include 20 minerals, 13 vitamins, 11 essential amino acids and 2 essential fatty acids. When these essential elements are missing from the human diet, the immune system falters and health deteriorates. Consume healing foods as part of your immune system cure, and be sure to include as many of them as possible on a daily basis. Remember, to keep your immune system performing at its peak, you must eat 7 to 10 half-cup servings of fruits and/or vegetables every day.

FATS THAT HEAL, FATS THAT KILL

Yes, there are fats that can kill you and most of us eat them every day. And no, not all fats are bad. Although it is true that fats are associated with cancer, arthritis, heart disease and diabetes, it is not all fat, but bad fats that are the culprits. Some fats have powerful healing properties.

Another problem with fat occurs when good fats are changed into bad fats. This is what happens when seeds and nuts are processed into the oils, margarines and shortenings we buy at the supermarket— every essential nutrient is removed or destroyed. Through this process, the fat molecules are also altered into disease-causing molecules, making them not only unusable by the body, but ultimately toxic.

Low-Fat Diets are Killing Us

Low-fat diets are not going to protect you from disease. Researchers found that women who live in Spain, Greece and Italy have very low rates of breast cancer compared to women living in the United States, even though the former consume 50 percent of their diet from fats. It is the *type* of fat that is important. These women were consuming fat in the form of cold-pressed, extra-virgin olive oil.

Certain indigenous peoples, the Inuit especially, eat approximately 60 percent of their diet from fats and yet they have the lowest rates of arteriosclerosis, cancer and diabetes. The reason for this is that the fats that they eat are rich in health-protective essential fatty acids. Standard American Diets (SAD) and diets consumed by other affluent nations are made up of approximately 40 percent fat. This SAD diet is essential fatty acid deficient and, as a result, does not provide disease protection.

Slick marketing techniques have convinced many North Americans that "caffeine-free," "cholesterol-free," "sugar-free" and "no fat" means healthy. ("Sugar-free" usually means replaced with toxic aspartame.) Today, you are not sold a product for all the benefits it contains, but more often for what it lacks. The process to remove healthy ingredients from foods frequently leaves us with a chemically altered toxic soup of ingredients. Patrick and I would rather our children ate a small amount of real sugar than sugar substitutes. We taught them to read the label of the food they are eating. If they couldn't pronounce the ingredients, then it probably was not safe to eat the food.

The Guise of Cholesterol-free

"Cholesterol-free" is a term used on almost every non-animal product. We laugh when we see "cholesterol-free" on products that never contained cholesterol in the first place. Labeling a product this way is marketing hype that fools consumers into believing that if the product does not contain cholesterol, it must be healthy.

We will look at the cholesterol story later. Suffice it to say, healing fats do not increase cholesterol; they decrease it. It is oxidized cholesterol found in packaged foods that is the problem. Foods such as powdered milk and eggs, packaged meats, bread-machine bread mixes, cake mixes and crackers, to name a few, are full of oxidized cholesterol. Eggs and butter are not the villains they are made out to be. A lack of fruits and vegetables in the diet are the main reason that cholesterol gets out of hand. The fiber found in fruits and vegetables is essential in keeping cholesterol in check. Oxidized cholesterol also occurs in the body when inadequate amounts of the antioxidant nutrients are provided. Eliminate packaged foods as much as possible, and if you must eat them, supplement your diet with the extra antioxidants discussed in chapter 3.

What Are Essential Fats?

Research shows that essential fatty acids and the minor ingredients sterols and sterolins from flaxseed oil and olive oil are effective at boosting the immune system when used in combination with a plant-based diet. Essential fatty acids include omega 3 (alpha-linolenic acid) and omega 6 (linoleic acid). From these essential fatty acids other important derivatives called prostaglandins are made in the human body. On a moment-to-moment basis, essential fatty acids are used to regulate cellular activity. The immune system requires essential fatty acids to help fight infections, yeast and bacteria. Essential fatty acids are required for the body's production of tumor necrosis factor. As discussed earlier, TNK produced by the immune system is effective at destroying cancerous cells. Several essential fatty acid derivatives also have anti-tumor effects.

Prostaglandins, hormone-like substances made from essential fatty acids, can be either beneficial or harmful to the body depending on what type of foods you eat. If you eat plenty of flaxseed or olive oil, your prostaglandins will keep PMS at bay and inflammation under control. On the other hand,

Types of Fats

Saturated fats	Saturated fats are semi-solid at room temperature. Sources of saturated fats are animal fats (red meat, pork, lamb), dairy products and tropical oils (coconut, palm). These fatty acids are associated with LDL "bad" cholesterol.
Monounsaturated fats	Monounsaturated fats remain liquid at room temperature; they solidify with cold temperatures. Sources of these fatty acids are olive, canola and peanut oils. These fatty acids are associated with HDL "good" cholesterol.
Polyunsaturated fats	Polyunsaturated fats, which are omega-6 fats, remain liquid at room temperature and stay in that form at colder temperatures. Sources of polyunsaturated fats are corn, safflower, sesame, soy and sunflower oils.
Superunsaturated fats	Superunsaturated fats are even more liquid at room temperature, and don't solidify unless frozen. The freezing point is lower than omega-6 oils. These fats include omega-3 essential fatty acids from flax and fish.

if you eat too much saturated fat from red meat, pork, lamb, beef and other animal products, dairy or tropical fats (palm and coconut oil), inflammatory reactions as seen in arthritis and fibromyalgia may result. Prostaglandins can be your friend or foe depending on the type of fats you eat.

Fat Processing and Cooking is the Killer

Don't eat refined, processed fats, the ones found in supermarket oils. They have been damaged through the process of deodorization, making them colorless, odorless and tasteless; they have been treated with a corrosive

Will New Margarine Be Healthier?

A *Vancouver Sun* report, July 22, 1998, states: "Cholesterol-reducing margarine is on the way." A margarine especially made to reduce cholesterol is headed for North American shelves in early 1999. Studies have shown that it works by preventing the body from absorbing dietary cholesterol and inhibiting the liver's own production of cholesterol.

McNeil Consumer Products will supply the ingredient called sitostanol which is made from sitosterol derived from pine trees. Scientists predict that sitostanol can be used in foods from salad dressing to ice cream. But should we trust them? Remember, these scientists also told us that margarine and vegetable oils would help us reduce heart disease and lower cholesterol. Then, over a decade later, a Harvard research study found that "risk of heart attack doubled, and cancer was linked to the increased consumption of margarines and hydrogenated oils and shortenings." Now scientists tell us that those same foods will lower cholesterol with sitostanol added to them.

For decades cardiac specialists have advised against the consumption of butter because they wrongfully believed it increased blood cholesterol and thereby cardiac disease. The culprit that raises cholesterol and causes heart disease is not butter; it is the trans-fatty acids found in hydrogenated margarines, cooking oils and most packaged foods.

sodium hydroxide, then with phosphoric acid; then they are bleached and heated to frying temperature—all this to extend shelf-life.

Hydrogenation, a process used to turn liquid oils into a solid to make margarines, shortenings and partially hydrogenated vegetable oils, changes the shape of the oil molecules, rendering them toxic to the body. Trans-fatty acids are a result of this process and a bane of our existence.

"Cholesterol-free, no fat, fake fat and light" are marketing tools used by major food manufacturers to encourage consumers to buy their products. Counting fat grams has become a national pastime. Unfortunately, people believe that by monitoring the amount of fat in their food, they are reducing their risk of heart disease and cancer, and managing their weight. As mentioned earlier, the problem is not fat in general—it is the type of fat and the way it has been processed.

Canada's food-labeling regulations offer little protection to consumers. While all packaged foods must have a list of ingredients, manufacturers are not required to provide information about processing, damage and certain nutrients—such as the amount of fat, fiber or iron a product contains, unless they are making a specific health claim. When a food is promoted as low fat or fat-free, the label must declare the amount of fat the food contains. Even with careful reading, however, consumers remain unaware of one of the most harmful forms of fat that slips through the labeling criteria—trans-fatty acids. This dangerous fat is formed when liquid vegetable oils are hardened into solid fats, a process that extends a product's shelf-life. Trans-fatty acids increase the risk of heart disease by raising LDL, the "bad" form of cholesterol, and total cholesterol. Most products touted as cholesterol-free are high in trans-fatty acids and are linked to increases in heart disease rates. It is dangerously ironic that the foods people are using to lower their risk of heart disease actually cause it. Although margarine and other fat-reduced products are being increasingly consumed, heart disease rates are not decreasing.

Check the next product you purchase for its fat content. Add up the percentages of saturated, monounsaturated and polyunsaturated fats it contains. Most likely, when these percentages are totaled, they do not equal 100 percent. See if trans-fatty acids are listed—they are generally the missing percentage. Regardless of any added ingredients or health benefits, products that contain trans-fatty acids cannot be health promoting. They are proven to cause cancer, obesity and heart disease.

There is no nutritional substance as controversial as cholesterol, and no substance about which there is more confusion. The fact is, 999 out of

1,000 people can control their cholesterol levels with simple dietary changes alone. Cholesterol is essential to our health, which means that our body has to manufacture it in order to keep us alive. For 70 percent of the population, an increase in the consumption of cholesterol decreases production within the body by means of a protective, regulating feedback system. The other 30 percent may have to limit cholesterol consumption through dietary manipulation. Do not consume foods that contain trans-fatty acids or have been hydrogenated and look for unrefined organic seed oils in the refrigerator section of your health food store. Relax, butter is fine in moderation, especially if you have made sure to get optimal amounts of the ESA's omega-3 and omega-6.

The American Heart Association states that the average American eats almost 60 pounds of fat per year. Even though there has been a reduction in fat consumption over the last ten years by approximately 7 percent, heart disease and especially obesity are still on the rise. Those who live to count fat grams and percentages of fat will want to know how much fat is acceptable. Approximately 30 percent of your diet can be made up of the healing fats we mention below eaten in conjunction with a healthy diet.

Hydrogenated foods such as margarine, shortening and all partially hydrogenated oils:

- cause heart disease;
- increase LDL—the "bad" cholesterol—and lower HDL—the "good" cholesterol;
- increase inflammatory responses;
- cause toxicity in the liver;
- raise cholesterol levels;
- promote aging and free radical damage; and
- inhibit immune function.

Better Butter Recipe

Take one pound of butter and blend in a food processor with one cup of organic unrefined seed oil blend. Mix until smooth. Put in a sealed container and refrigerate. This better butter will be ready to spread soft from the refrigerator, and is rich in essential fatty acids.

Frying, especially deep-frying, causes fat molecules to form free radicals, which are destructive to health. Blackened or barbecued foods are also full of free radicals. Reduce them or, better yet, eliminate them from your diet. If you must eat them, be sure to supplement your diet with plenty of antioxidants, vitamins A, C, E and zinc and selenium. Double the daily dosage recommended in chapter 3 to protect you against potential cancers.

Reduce your red meat consumption. The American Cancer Society recommends cutting out all red meat to prevent cancer. A study published in the *Journal of the National Cancer Society* found that men who ate meat 4 to 5 times a week had 4 times more risk of developing colon cancer as men who ate meat once a month. The study also showed that if they ate lean meat, their risk of prostate cancer was twice that of non-meat eaters.

Saturated fat consumption, either through eating red meat or processed meats such as hot dogs and luncheon meats, increase your risk of cancer. A troubling study by researchers at the University of Southern California School of Medicine, reported in the June 1995 issue of *Cancer Causes and Control*, found that hot dogs were the culprit in the higher incidence of leukemia among 232 children in Los Angeles. The children, 10 years and under, with leukemia were matched with a control group of children who were healthy. Those with the highest incidence of leukemia regularly ate more than 12 hot dogs each month. Two other reports published in the same issue found that children born to mothers who eat just one hot dog weekly during pregnancy or fathers who ate hot dogs regularly before conception have double the normal risk of developing brain tumors. The researchers suggest that the trigger for the cancer is the buildup of highly carcinogenic nitrosamines, metabolites of nitrates used to preserve processed meats, including hot dogs.

Eating red meat also aggravates conditions such as multiple sclerosis and arthritis. Arachidonic acid, a substance which is found in red meats, is linked to an increase in pro-inflammatory factors. Simply removing red meat from the diets of individuals suffering from arthritis can eliminate painful symptoms.

In addition to including the protective fats in your diet, you should eliminate the killer fats. Check your kitchen pantry and throw away any supermarket cooking oils, except extra-virgin olive oil. Purchase your oils in light protective packaging, cold pressed and preferably organic. Check the packaged food you have and look for the words "hydrogenated" or "partially hydrogenated" and throw away these foods as well. Stop buying red meat, processed meats, especially hot dogs, and reach for lean poultry, fatty, cold-water fish and tofu dogs.

Health-Protective Fats

Protective fats are found in seeds and nuts and their unrefined, cold-pressed oils, fatty fish, avocados, whole grains, dark green vegetables and olives. These essential fatty acid–rich foods are cancer protective. Flaxseed is especially rich in essential fatty acids but should be balanced with EFA's from sunflower and sesame seeds or oils. It also contains important phytonutrients that have been shown to have anticancer effects. Lignans are one phytonutrient that is found in high concentrations in flaxseeds.

Lignans have been proven to have anticancer, antifungal, antibacterial and antiviral properties. Flaxseeds contain more lignans than any other plant. Ground flaxseed contains seven more lignans than the oil, and also provides an excellent source of fiber. Add at least one tablespoon of ground flaxseed to your diet. Use a portable coffee grinder and only grind what you are going to eat. You don't want the seed to lose its valuable ingredients due to oxidation.

Lignans are only one of several phytonutrients found in seeds and nuts; these include carotene and beta-sitosterol and its glucoside beta-sitosterolin. When nuts and seeds are made into colorless, odorless, tasteless oils, the beta-sitosterol and beta-sitosterolin are removed as they give oils a cloudy look which food manufacturers dislike. Processing these phytonutrients out of foods is unfortunate, since they are important immune enhancers in the fight against cancer. Research using Sterinol found that plant fats act to promote the formation of other healthy fatty acids from linoleic acid. These fatty acids are needed to make prostaglandins, important in all cell-mediated immune functions (see chapter 2).

Eat at least 1 to 2 tablespoons of essential fatty acid-rich oil per day and eat 1 tablespoon of ground flaxseeds and sunflower seeds along with 3 capsules of Sterinol as well. Look for organic, cold-pressed oils, and remember, if the oil is clear and colorless, it has been refined. Don't buy it. Udo's Choice oil and Omega Balance are the two oils we use in our kitchens. Omega Nutrition (see Appendix I) also has a wonderful pumpkin spread and healthy culinary oils. Look in Appendix II for a supplier near you.

GENETICALLY ENGINEERED FOODS

Genes found in each cell of an organism determine its characteristics and biological attributes. Certain genes determine whether you will have brown eyes or blue, whether a rat will have white hair or gray, whether a flower will have five petals or four, and whether the protein content of a seed will be great or small. They provide the building blocks of life.

Genetically engineered foods are foods that have had their genetic blueprint altered by a technological process. Through this process, genes are either removed from their chain or inserted in another location in the chain—a process that could never have occurred in nature. Biotechnology labs, under pressure from giant food manufacturers, are searching for methods to keep foods from spoiling, to make them resistant to pests and to give them a better appearance—hence, genetic engineering.

We have been using a form of gene alteration for years, by selective breeding and combining certain plants to enhance particular traits. This has been accomplished, however, by using the plant's reproductive processes, not by totally rearranging the genetic code.

With the introduction of genetic engineering, scientists are now transferring genes between dissimilar species as well as infecting the target plant with foreign genes. Common examples of this include inserting fish genes into a tomato, and virus genes into a potato. Distorting the genetic code creates a mutant variation. Foods that go through this process are radically altered, the ramifications of which we may not realize for decades. In other words, humans are the experimental subjects to be tested. We are unaware of the side effects of genetically engineered foods. Already, scientists who oppose the alteration of our food source suspect that our immune system function could be seriously altered and allergies to these unusual foods may occur.

Altering foods so that they don't rot, won't grow mold or so that bugs will not even touch them may have long-term health implications that we should try to avoid. Choosing organic is one way of ensuring that you are not eating foods grown from the seeds of genetically engineered foods.

PLANTS PROVIDE GREAT DISEASE PROTECTION

The immune system cure is founded on the fact that fruits, vegetables, nuts, seeds, legumes, grains and sea vegetables are foods that heal. Eat plenty of them, whole, fresh and, whenever possible, organically grown. Plant foods contain phytonutrients, powerful immune system protectors. The foods we recommend are rich in phytonutrients, vitamins, minerals, amino acids and other important factors. Foods such as garlic and onions, yogurt, cruciferous vegetables, seeds and nuts, as well as fresh fish should be the foundation upon which you add a few important immune-enhancing food supplements.

Killer fats must be eliminated for the immune system cure diet to be effective. We can not emphasize this enough. Reducing the toxic burden on your immune system is the first step to supercharged immunity.

Free Radicals Beware: Garlic Present

Certain foods are especially valuable in boosting the immune system and preventing disease. Garlic is one food that has potent healing properties. More than 2,500 scientific published papers have extolled the virtues of this traditional food, also called an herb. Garlic has endured 5,000 years as a treatment for everything from the common cold to reptile bites. Current research focuses on garlic's antifungal, antiviral, anti-inflammatory, anticancer and antibacterial properties used in the treatment of asthma, heart disease, colds and flu, ear infections and diabetes. *Clinical Pearls*, summaries of nutritional medicine papers, reported on 20 studies that evaluated the protective effects of onions and garlic. Eight of these studies looked at the cancer-protective effects of garlic. In 19 of the 20 studies, onions and garlic were found to have a protective effect against gastrointestinal tract cancers. Researchers believed that the antibacterial and antimutagenic effects of these vegetables are the reasons for the anticancer effect.

Garlic contains more than 200 compounds including sulfur and trace minerals. Much of the information available to consumers on the benefits of garlic focuses on the compound allicin, but as in most foods, garlic's powerful effect is most likely due to many factors, not just one. The sulfur compounds found in garlic are the basis for its immune-enhancing capabilities. Sulfur is an effective free radical scavenger with super-antioxidant properties. Although it is most often examined for its protective effects against heart disease, for the purposes of the immune system cure, we will focus on garlic's ability to boost immune function.

Sulfur enhances the function of natural killer cells, thereby boosting the immune system's ability to fight cancerous cells and cells infected by bacteria and viruses. Garlic is well known for its stomach cancer protective effects. Moreover, garlic contains selenium and, as discussed in chapter 3, selenium is one of the top ten immune-boosting nutrients. What is most interesting is garlic's ability to help the body detoxify heavy metals, especially mercury. Heavy metal toxicity is a serious burden to the immune system.

In cases where an individual has become resistant to antibiotic therapy, garlic, with its powerful antiviral, antibacterial, antifungal activity, is a proven alternative.

Add fresh garlic to your diet, but if you can't tolerate it, take a garlic capsule daily. Also eat plenty of onions, as they contain quercetin, a powerful flavonoid discussed in chapter 4.

Cancer Protection from Cruciferous Vegetables

Consume the following cruciferous vegetables as often as possible, either steamed, in soups or lightly sautéed on low heat: broccoli, cabbage, cauliflower, bok choy, collard greens, rutabaga, kale, daikon and salad radishes, mustard greens, turnips and watercress. These vegetables have been shown to slow colon cancer growth and reduce intestinal polyps. They also reduce breast cancer rates by helping to eliminate excess estrogens from the body. Cruciferous vegetables were the first to be promoted by the American Cancer Society as cancer preventive. These vegetables also increased levels of glutathione, and as we discovered in chapter 3, glutathione is extremely important as a generator of immune cells and as a powerful detoxifier that eliminates carcinogens. Low levels of gluthione are associated with early aging and even death.

Broccoli contains sulphoraphane, a powerful phytonutrient that stimulates certain enzymes to deactivate cancer cells, allowing them to be digested and eliminated from the body. Cancer cells are often ignored by the immune system as foreign invaders, and as a result, they are allowed to set up house. Sulphoraphane helps turn on helper T-cells to recognize them as invaders and tell killer cells to respond and destroy.

Broccoli sprouts have more than ten times the sulphoraphane as mature broccoli spears. Sprouting cruciferous vegetables is one way of getting the maximum benefit from the plants. Do not buy grocery store ready-to-eat sprouts as they are suspected of being contaminated with salmonella. We sprout at home in a jar on the kitchen windowsill.

How to Sprout at Home

Sprouts are an excellent source of greens that can be grown year-round. They are especially important during the winter months when fresh greens are expensive and difficult to find.

To sprout at home, you will need a one-quart (1-liter) canning jar, cheesecloth, netting or a clean piece of pantyhose to cover the opening of the jar, and a canning ring or rubber band to secure the fabric.

Buy organic seeds including alfalfa, mung beans, lentils, sunflower or wheat berries. These are the easiest to sprout.

For each one-quart (1-liter) canning jar, you will need:

  3 tablespoons of alfalfa seeds—takes 5 to 7 days to mature

  1 cup mung beans or lentils—takes 3 to 4 days to mature

  1 cup hulled sunflower seeds or wheat berries—takes 3 to 4 days to mature

Sprout on your kitchen countertop, not in direct full sunlight, at room temperature.

Place the required amount of seeds in the jar. Add 4 times the amount of purified water as seeds (i.e., 1 cup of seeds needs 4 cups of water). Cover the opening of the jar with cloth and secure with a rubber band or canning ring. Let the seeds soak for 12 hours, drain all the water and place the jar upside down on a drainer for 5 minutes. Place the jar on a slant with the opening down. Don't let the sprouts dry out; they should be rinsed in the morning, at dinnertime and before you go to bed. To rinse them, fill the jar with water and let the sprouts soak up the water for 5 minutes. Drain and return to the slanted position. Follow the sprouting times above, and on the last day place the sprouts on a brightly lit windowsill so they can mature, increasing their chlorophyll and vitamin D content. Sprouts must be kept in the refrigerator and eaten within several days. Remember to grow more sprouts so you always have a ready supply.

Much-Maligned Avocado

Avocados have been given a bad rap. Physicians have been warning heart patients and those on weight reduction diets to avoid the avocado. Superhero of the immune system, avocado is rich in the powerful detoxifier glutathione. Glutathione-rich avocados actually help clean the body of dangerous oxidized fats. Wrongly, avocado has been dismissed as a healing food due to its fat content, but it contains monounsaturated fats, the ones we recommend to help the body deal with oxidation and free radicals. Potassium and chromium are also found in avocados. Potassium is used to treat high blood pressure, water balance in the body, and kidney, heart and adrenal function. Chromium works to help control blood sugar levels by helping insulin work more efficiently. It is used for the treatment of hypoglycemia and diabetes, high cholesterol and to normalize triglyceride levels and to increase fat loss.

Tomatoes Rich in Lycopene

You will hear more and more about the tomato in the next few years. After examining certain nationalities for incidence of cancer, researchers found that Italians, who eat more tomatoes on average than any other group, have lower rates of cancer. Tomatoes are rich in the carotenoid lycopene, a phytonutrient also found in watermelon and grapefruit. It is an oil-soluble phytonutrient with powerful anticancer and prostate protective properties. The lycopene found in tomatoes is better absorbed when they are eaten with oil. Pour a little flaxseed or olive oil on your tomato salad or add these oils to your tomato sauce just before you serve it, and you will absorb up to 70 percent of the lycopene. (See chapter 4 for more information about carotenoids.)

Immune-Boosting Fruits

Certain fruits are packed with immune-boosting anticancer ingredients. Choose dark-colored fruits. The dark pigments they contain have the highest levels of antioxidants and phytonutrients. Berries, especially cranberries, blueberries, bilberries, raspberries and strawberries, are packed with potent phytonutrients and antioxidants. Cranberries and blueberries contain anthocyanins with powerful antioxidant and free radical scavenging activity.

They also inhibit bacteria from attaching to the wall of the bladder, thereby stopping urinary tract infections. Make vitamin C–rich berries a staple in your daily diet.

Grapes contain more than a dozen known antioxidants, as well as reservatrol, a phytonutrient shown to have cancer-protective effects. They also contain ellagic acid, selenium and quercetin, a powerful flavonoid mentioned in chapter 4. Red and purple grapes and their juice are richer in antioxidants than green grapes. Research shows that grapes may put small tumors into remission and enhance natural killer cell activity. They inhibit oxidation, unclog arteries and reduce cholesterol, fight allergies and have anti-inflammatory properties. An extract from the grape seed, proanthocyanidin oligomers (PCO), has also shown immune-enhancing, anticancer effects. The move toward growing grapes engineered to contain no seeds is a negative assault on the food chain.

If you choose a PCO supplement, take at least 100 mg per day. For severe allergic reactions, take up to 500 mg per day until symptoms abate.

Ellagic acid is a naturally occurring polyphenol that has powerful anti-mutagenic and anticancer properties. Grapes, strawberries, raspberries, black currants and walnuts are good food sources of ellagic acid. Strawberries have been shown to have a protective effect against prostate cancer which scientists believe is due to the ellagic acid content of the fruit.

Eat plenty of fresh, preferably organic, phytonutrient-rich fruits such as watermelons, lemons, limes, oranges, grapes with the seed and grapefruit. Citrus fruits, especially oranges, are packed with carotenoids, flavonoids and vitamin C. Grapefruit, rich in lycopene, is also a good source of glutathione, the immune system master nutrient.

VEGETARIANS:

- have more voracious immune cells
- have lower rates of cancer
- have reduced breast and ovarian cancers
- have less heart disease
- live, on average, ten years longer than red-meat eaters
- are 40 percent less likely to die of cancer
- have lower rates of Type II diabetes

People who eat plenty of fresh fruits and vegetables have stellar immune systems that are able to ward off disease more effectively, and if they succumb to cancer they recover faster.

Although we are not recommending a vegetarian diet, the facts shown above are very interesting.

KILLER SUGAR

On average, North Americans eat 125 pounds of sugar annually in the form of baked goods, soft drinks, bread spreads, alcohol, beer, catsup, salad dressings and sweeteners. Sugar is at the root of so many problems, it should be sold with a warning that says: Sugar can increase your risk of developing cancer, heart disease, varicose veins, kidney disorders, arthritis, diabetes, obesity, migraine headaches and high blood pressure, to name a few. Our immune system function is severely hampered by sugar consumption.

One study evaluated the ability of immune cells to engulf bacteria. The study looked at five groups of subjects. Group one was the control group; the second group consumed 6 teaspoons of sugar; and the third, fourth and fifth groups consumed 12, 18 and 24 teaspoons of sugar, respectively. Over five hours, blood samples were extracted and mixed with bacteria. Immune cells in the control group ate approximately 14 bacteria. With each consecutive group, the number of bacteria eaten was reduced until, in the group that consumed 24 teaspoons of sugar, only one bacteria was destroyed. Immune suppression was seen well after consumption of the sugar. The message: eliminate sugar from your diet as much as possible. Concentrated fruit juices are also a high source of sugar, so make sure that your children are not drinking excessive amounts.

The negative effects of sugar consumption have been well documented in medical journals around the world. Sugar is the culprit in increasing the risk of contracting certain cancers, especially of the breast and colon. It causes heart disease, raises triglycerides and blood pressure, lowers the body's production of antibodies, causes macrophages to be inactive, increases infection rate in diabetics and causes deficiencies in B vitamins, chromium, copper and molybdenum. Most important, sugar reduces immunity.

When they are under the influence of sugar, immune cells are unable to march around the body fighting invaders. A form of paralysis takes place and these cells are rendered ineffective. Sugar also increases the growth of

Candida albicans, a yeast organism responsible for poor nutrient absorption, chronic fatigue, depression, weight gain and digestive upsets. One teaspoon of white sugar can devastate your immune system for up to six hours, leaving you vulnerable to attack from viruses, bacteria, cancer cells and parasites.

Natural sugars as found in foods are not as devastating when consumed in the whole food form. For example, sugar in the form of the whole apple is better than the juice of the apple without the fiber. Similarly, a whole carrot is much better than only the juice of the carrot. Sugar from concentrated juice, maple syrup, rice syrup, barley malt, honey and beets are only slightly better than table sugar in reducing a negative immune response, increasing cholesterol and triglycerides. Whole foods with their natural sugars are the best choice. Never chose aspartame or other artificial sweeteners as they are toxic. Aspartame rapidly turns into dangerous formaldehyde in the body. If you only have a choice between sugar-sweetened foods and aspartame under the trademark NutraSweet, choose sugar. Even with all the problems related to sugar consumption it is nowhere near as toxic as aspartame.

If you have serious sugar cravings, talk to a naturopathic doctor about treating you for *Candida albicans* yeast overgrowth. You may also want to supplement your diet with 100 to 200 mcg of chromium picolinate per day as it helps to reduce cravings for sugar.

If your children are ill and must take antibiotics, ask the pharmacist to prepare the liquid carrier without sugar or aspartame. Since sugar reduces the immune system's effectiveness, it definitely should not be added to an antibiotic.

Everyone needs a little sweet once in a while, but try choosing apple crisp over pecan pie, or make sauces with pureed fruits without sugar. Examine the amount of sugar you consume in a day. You will likely be very surprised.

EATING TOO MUCH DEPRESSES IMMUNITY

Overeating suppresses the immune system. Tests performed by the National Institutes on Aging, Bethesda, Maryland, revealed that when animals were fed 50 percent less calories per day, their immune response was enhanced, thymus size was maintained and T-cell function improved. Although this study looked at high calorie consumption, it did not distinguish what types of calories were consumed. Heavy meat-based or sugar-laden foods would definitely have a negative impact on immune function, whereas calories in the form of fruits, vegetables, legumes, nuts and seeds would boost immunity. Moreover, since even an additional 20 pounds can lower your immunity, weight management is an important aspect of maintaining a peak operating immune system.

YOGURT: SUPER-IMMUNE BOOSTER

Keeping the immune system in prime operating order has never before been so important. With today's antibiotic-resistant bacteria and virulent viruses, we must provide the body with the proper defenses. Poor nutritional choices and an overprescribing of antibiotics have weakened the body's ability to attack and destroy potential disease-causing bacteria, parasites and viruses. Probiotics, including *lactobacillus acidophilus*, *lactobacillus bulgaricus* and *bifidobacterium bifidum* found in a healthy digestive tract, are a few of the important microorganisms that we can use to enhance immunity. Ongoing research confirms the benefits of supplementing the diet with probiotics. The following are just a few examples.

In his research, Dr. Khem Shahani has shown that probiotics, especially lactobacillus acidophilus DDS-1, enhance immune function by eliminating or inhibiting the formation of cancer-causing chemicals. Nitrates, commonly used in food processing, can be converted via enzymes to carcinogenic nitrosamines in the gut. Lactobacillus acidophilus is able to halt this process first by reducing the quantity of potential carcinogens, and second by deactivating certain cancer-causing enzymes, especially d-glucuronidase and b-glucosidase.

The "Benefits of Yogurt," a report published in the *Journal of Immunotherapy*, found that acidophilus containing yogurt eaten over several months increased gamma-interferon, an important immune-enhancing protein that prevents viruses from reproducing themselves. Also noted was a reduction in inflammatory responses of the gut. IgE, an immunoglobulin that is effective in destroying parasites, is enhanced when lactobacillus bulgaricus was added to the diet. It was found to have powerful antibacterial properties, allowing IgE to function optimally.

Another study involving 21 female patients between the ages of 40 and 75 undergoing radiation for the treatment of cervical or uterine cancer were given yogurt containing friendly bacteria. (Friendly bacteria maintain a healthy gastrointestinal tract, immune system and nutritional status. Two of the most important friendly bacteria include lactobacillus acidophilus and bifidobacterium bifidum. There are also "bad" bacteria that colonize the gut, causing disease.) A significant reduction in radiation-induced diarrhea was seen, as well as a general improvement in overall well-being. Diarrhea is a serious complication of cancer therapies, causing weight loss, immune depression and nutritional deficiencies. Worldwide, diarrhea is a major cause of death in young children and an annoyance for travelers. By restoring balance to the intestinal tract, probiotics are a fast, effective remedy, often eliminating the condition within several days.

Yogurt is a super-immune-enhancing food. It contains calcium D-glucarate that helps metabolize excess estrogen to be eliminated from the body via the liver. Excess estrogens are thought to be a factor in the promotion of breast cancer. Adding yogurt to your diet may have a protective effect against the disease. While we are waiting for research to confirm these claims, simply adding one cup of yogurt to your daily diet, along with the super-immune-boosting foods we have been discussing, may be an easy way to prevent disease.

Lactobacillus acidophilus is also able to concentrate selenium in cells. We are well aware of the benefits of selenium in inhibiting certain cancers, especially breast cancer. It is known that in areas where soil selenium levels are low, certain cancers are high. The importance of keeping intracellular selenium levels high cannot be understated. With the simple addition of probiotic supplements, along with selenium, this can be accomplished.

Adding one cup of probiotic-rich yogurt to your diet daily will enhance your immune function. If you cannot accomplish this or you don't like yogurt, take probiotic supplements as recommended on the label. We recommend Klaire Laboratories Vital Life probiotics or Natren probiotics.

HOW CAN I EAT ENOUGH GREENS?

How can I eat 7 to 10 half-cup servings of fruits and vegetables per day? you might ask. Eat as many as you can and supplement with freshly squeezed juices and green drinks (see below). Juicing several fruits or vegetables will provide your body with plenty of phytonutrients, especially sterols and sterolins, but it won't supply you with the fiber you need unless you add the fiber left over from juicing to recipes such as quick breads and muffins.

However, as mentioned above, you may consume too much sugar in juices, so limit your consumption to one glass per day. Drink it immediately after juicing and "chew" it to start the digestive process. (Chewing your juice allows the salivary enzymes found in your saliva to begin the digestive process. Drink a small amount of juice and chew it, with your mouth closed, for a few seconds before swallowing.) Many of the phytonutrients are destroyed if left too long exposed to the air.

FABULOUS FIBER

Fiber is essential to maintaining cholesterol levels and eliminating toxins by way of the bowel. Good bowel movements at least once a day are essential for a healthy immune system. One doctor said that he stopped asking people if they were regular because they always said yes. They thought that regular meant once a week. If you are not having a good bowel movement at least once a day, you are constipated and your body has to deal with too many toxins. In his lectures, Udo Erasmus tells people they must have one 12-inch bowel movement, or three, 4-inch bowel movements, each day to stay in top form. The bowel movement must also float, which means it contains plenty of fiber.

Eat at least 40 grams of fiber-rich foods daily. There are two types of fiber, soluble and insoluble. Insoluble fiber is found in grains such as bran, as well as psyllium husk. Soluble fiber is found in apples in the form of pectin, the gooey stuff in cooked oatmeal and the slippery substance

Benefits of Fiber

- Insoluble fiber acts as a bulking agent to speed elimination.
- Soluble fiber binds to excess cholesterol, allowing it to be eliminated.
- Fiber-rich foods make you feel full and can help manage your weight.
- Fiber helps regulate blood sugar levels.
- Bowel toxins are excreted faster when fiber-rich foods are consumed regularly.

surrounding flaxseeds that have been soaked. Don't forget that nuts and seeds are excellent fiber-rich foods. Brazil nuts in the shell not only provide fiber but are also rich in sterols and sterolins and selenium, which are all-important to a healthy defense system. Ground flaxseed is Lorna's favorite fiber food, added to cereal in the morning or cooked into a delicious pudding! Flax is truly one great food.

GREENS IN A GLASS

Green drinks are a good source of many phytonutrients and fiber, in a quick, easy-to-use form. These super food drinks contain ingredients such as alfalfa, wheat grass, barley, brown rice germ, sprouted grains and soy, spirulina, dulse, chlorella, probiotics, bee pollen, milk thistle, green tea, grape seeds, Siberian ginseng, licorice root, ginkgo biloba, bilberry and phosphatidyl choline. Most super food drinks contain an assortment of the above ingredients for a convenient drink to supplement a normal diet rich in fruits and vegetables. These drinks are excellent for people on the run and for teenagers. Consumed straight up or mixed with organic fruit juices or blended into a power shake, they are a great way to get your greens fast. Every emergency kit, hiking pack or travel bag should not be without a ready supply of greens. GREENS+, Udo's Beyond Greens, and Green Alive are some of the recommended green drinks (see Appendix I).

PROTEIN FOR REPAIR

Nuts, seeds, legumes, fresh fish and free-range poultry, dairy products and eggs provide us with the amino acids necessary for protein production. There are 20 amino acids, of which 12 can be made by the body. This leaves us with 8 essential amino acids that we must get from our food. Protein is required for cellular repair and to manufacture CP-450, an important protective enzyme. Adequate levels of CP-450 have been shown to decrease breast cancer risk and it also acts as a free radical scavenger. Protein deficiency can result in a depressed immune system.

If you are a fitness enthusiast or do heavy physical labor, you will have higher protein requirements than the couch potato. On average, it is recommended that people eat 3 to 4 ounces of protein from the sources mentioned above, or make protein consumption approximately 15 to 20 percent of your diet. Choose free-range chicken and eggs and wild fish over farm-grown. Purchase nuts in the shell and buy organic legumes if possible. For those with blood sugar problems, dividing your protein into small portions eaten throughout the day will aid in controlling symptoms.

Acid/alkaline effects of food are important. High-protein diets create an acid environment in the body. Acid-creating diets have been linked to increased risk of cancer, especially stomach cancer, and they are also associated with depressed immunity. Choose approximately 75 percent of your foods from the alkalizing foods listed below and the rest from the acidifying foods choices.

Acidifying and Alkalizing Foods

A RECIPE FOR LIFE

This chart provides information that shows the contribution of various food substances to the acidifying or alkalizing of body fluids and, ultimately, to the urine, saliva, and venous blood.

In general, it is important to eat a diet that contains foods from both sides of the chart. Allergic reactions and other forms of stress tend to produce acids in the body. The presence of high acidity indicates that more of your foods should be selected from the alkalizing group.

The kidneys help to maintain the neutrality of body fluids by excreting the excess acid or alkali in the urine. You may find it useful to check your urine pH using pHydrion paper in order to find out if your food selection is providing the desired balance. Check urine pH three times a day.

A urine pH of between 6.8 in the morning and 7.4 in the afternoon is ideal, but it will vary over the day depending upon the foods you eat as well as allergic reactions and other stress factors. Your urine pH should average 7.0.

People vary, but for most, the ideal diet is 75 percent alkalizing and 25 percent acidifying foods by volume.

ALKALIZING FOODS

Vegetables	Cucumber	Rutabaga
Garlic	*Eggplant	Sea Veggies
Asparagus	Kale	Spirulina (algae)
Fermented Veggies	Kohlrabi	Sprouts (all types)
Watercress	Lettuces (all types)	Squashes
Beets	Mushrooms	Alfalfa Grass
Broccoli	Mustard Greens	Barley Grass
Brussels Sprouts	Nova Scotia Dulse	Wheat Grass
Cabbage	Dandelions	Wild Greens
Carrot	Edible Flowers	
Cauliflower	Onions	
Celery	Parsnips (high-glycemic)	*Nightshade family foods
Chard	Peas	
Chlorella (algae)	*Peppers	Note: Use organically grown
Collard Greens	Pumpkin	whenever possible

ALKALIZING FOODS (continued)

Fruits
Apple
Apricot
Avocado
Banana (high-glycemic)
Blackberry
Blueberry
Cantaloupe
Cherries, Currants
Dates, Figs
Grapes
Grapefruit, Lime
Honeydew
Nectarine
Orange, Lemon
Peach, Pear
Pineapple
Raspberry (all berries)
Strawberry
Tangerine
*Tomato
Tropical Fruits
Watermelon

Protein
Free-Range Eggs
Whey Protein Powder
Fat-Free Cottage Cheese
Lean Chicken Breast
Organic Yogurt

Almonds
Chestnuts
Tofu (fermented)
Flax Seeds
Pumpkin Seeds
Tempeh (fermented)
Squash Seeds
Sunflower Seeds
Millet
Sprouted Seeds, Nuts

Other
Apple cider vinegar
Bee Pollen
Lecithin Granules
Dairy-Free Probiotic Cultures

Beverages
GREENS+
Veggie Juices
Fresh Fruit Juice (unsweetened)
Organic Milk (unpasteurized)
Mineral Water (non-carbonated)
Quality Water

Teas
Green Tea
Herbal Tea

Dandelion Tea
Ginseng
Bancha Tea
Kombucha

Sweeteners
Stevia

Spices & Seasonings
Cinnamon
Curry
Ginger
Mustard
Chili Peppers
Salt (Sea, Celtic)
Miso
Tamari
All Herbs

Oriental Vegetables
Maitake
Daikon
Dandelion Root
Shiitake
Kombu
Reishi
Nori
Umeboshi
Wakame
Sea Veggies

ACIDIFYING FOODS

Fats & Oils
Avocado Oil
Canola Oil
Corn Oil
Hemp Seed Oil
Flax Oil
Grape Seed Oil
Lard
Olive Oil
Safflower Oil
Sesame Oil
Sunflower Oil

Fruits
Cranberries

Grains
Rice Cakes
Wheat Cakes
Amaranth
Barley
Buckwheat

Corn
Oats (rolled)
Quinoa
Rice (Brown, Basmati)
Rye
Spelt
Kamut
Wheat
Hemp Seed Flour

Dairy, Milk & Hard Cheeses
Cheese, Cow
Cheese, Goat
Cheese, Processed
Cheese, Sheep
Milk
Butter

Nuts & Butters
Cashews
Filberts
Brazil Nuts

Peanuts
Peanut Butter
Pecans
Tahini
Walnuts

Animal Protein
Beef
Carp
Clams
Duck
Fish, White Meat
Lamb
Lobster
Mussels
Oysters
Pork
Rabbit
Salmon
Shrimp
Scallops
Tuna

ACIDIFYING FOODS *(continued)*

Turkey	Pesticides	Hard Liquor
Venison	Herbicides	Wine
Pasta (White)	**Sweets & Sweeteners**	**Beans & Legumes**
Noodles	Molasses	Black Beans
Macaroni	Candy	Chick Peas
Spaghetti	Honey	Green Peas
	Maple Syrup	Kidney Beans
Other	Saccharin	Lentils
Distilled Vinegar	Soft Drinks	Lima Beans
Brewers Yeast	Sugar	Pinto Beans
Wheat Germ	Aspartame	Red Beans
*Potatoes	Fruit-Flavored Drinks	Soybeans
		Soy Milk
Drugs & Chemicals	**Alcoholic Beverages**	White Beans
Drugs, Medicinal	Beer	Rice Milk
Drugs, Psychedelics	Spirits	Almond Milk

Soy: Good Protein Source

Soybeans are rich in protein, approximately 40 percent by volume. Soybeans contain natural plant estrogens called phytoestrogens, as well as genistein, which protects against breast and prostate cancer. Soy products are also rich in sterols and sterolins, enhance immunity, inhibit colon cancer in rats and halt colon cancer cells from reproducing. Soy products also help normalize estrogen and help to eliminate the hot flashes often associated with menopause.

Soy foods are easy to add to the diet. Simply crumble tofu into your favorite spaghetti sauce, or blend soft tofu into banana shakes. Drink soy milk instead of cow's milk. Tofu hot dogs and burgers are delicious and a great source of protein for everyone.

ARE YOU DIGESTING WHAT YOU EAT?

Good digestion is paramount to good health. If you are not digesting and absorbing what you eat, you are missing out on the benefits of your food. Take a good digestive enzyme supplement with each meal to ensure proper digestion. Your doctor can test you for a deficiency in hydrochloric acid (HCl), commonly known as stomach acid, which is required for optimal digestion. If you are low in HCl, symptoms such as gas and bloating will be present after eating.

We used to believe that low stomach acid was only a problem in the elderly, but it is now apparent that children are also affected. Diets high in refined foods decrease the body's need for hydrochloric acid, and refined foods do not contain their own enzymes which aid digestion. When you start adding whole, unrefined foods to your diet, include a digestive enzyme to give your body a running start at digestion.

PURE CLEAN WATER

Water, water, everywhere / nor any drop to drink. Clean, pure water is a hot commodity and by now, like most of us, we are sure you have added a water filtration system to your kitchen tap and shower spout. Chlorine, fluoride and chloramine are some of the toxic chemicals city water companies have added to our water in order to make it "safer" to drink. Microorganisms such as *Cryptosporidium oocysts* and *Giardia lamblia* are now common residents in our water due to clear-cut logging methods that upset the natural soil layer and cause these microorganisms to seep into the water supply. Synthetic solvents, herbicides, pesticides and plastic residues or hydrocarbons and inorganic metals are also found in the water we drink.

Deoxygenated water, as found in distilled water and bottled water, is a dead liquid and should not be consumed by humans. It is left with less than 1 mg of oxygen per liter and will not sustain life other than anaerobic organisms, a known danger to our health. Dead or deoxygenated water will also be searching for its charge and it will take it from you as necessary. (Molecules with a positive or negative charge such as water will search for the charge it requires. For example, this is why water molecules are drawn to one another when rain droplets form on a surface. They are seemingly pulled together to form a suspension.) Another reason not to choose distillation as a water purification process is that although many of the nasties found in water are removed, solvents are not removed, and they must be put through a carbon filter.

Aluminum in Water

Another problem with city water supplies is the aluminum sulfate that is used by water purification plants to remove impurities from the water. Alum, which gives water its distinct metal taste, is the key cause of neurological dysfunction. A ten-year study of approximately 3,777 people, aged 65, in 75 villages in southwest France, found that people who drink water containing 100 mcg of aluminum per liter double their risk of contracting Alzheimer's disease. Eight years into the study the team reported 200 more cases of Alzheimer's disease and 280 cases of senile dementia among those examined. Most cases occurred in the villages where water contained more than 100 mcg of aluminum per liter of water. Although the link between aluminum and Alzheimer's disease has not been clearly proven, the evidence is strong enough that we should try to avoid consuming it at all cost.

The best type of water filtration system combines a reverse-osmosis (RO) water system with a carbon filter (RO systems allow water to pass through a synthetic membrane that filters out contaminants); and to return oxygen to the water, use an ozone generator.

We recommend Vancouver Oxygen Research Technologies Ltd. for a home-use water ozonation system. See **www.oxygentechnologies.com** for more information.

GREEN TEA: YOUR COFFEE SUBSTITUTE

Although we commonly think of caffeine as only available in coffee, it is also found in chocolate bars, hot-chocolate drinks, soft drinks, decaffeinated coffee, iced tea and many over-the-counter medications such as Excedrin and Midol. Caffeine consumption can lead to high blood pressure, heart irregularities, sleep disturbances and fibroid breast cysts. Caffeine also causes magnesium to be excreted by the body. Considering that most North Americans are magnesium deficient, this is a serious side effect of caffeine consumption.

A can of cola contains approximately 30 to 40 mg of caffeine. We were surprised to learn that even decaffeinated coffee contains caffeine.

You may benefit by switching from coffee or other caffeinated beverages to herbal teas. There are many to choose from: dandelion, peppermint, licorice, chamomile, to name a few. Green tea, with its powerful immune-enhancing antioxidants, catechins and bioflavonoids, is an excellent hot beverage. Research shows that several cups of green tea each day have antiviral, anticancer and antibacterial effects. Look for organic green tea or choose a nutritional supplement made with green tea extract.

YOUR BODY HAS THE POWER TO HEAL

The immune system is designed to ward off disease, but it must be given the tools to accomplish the job. Eating a diet rich in organic fruits and vegetables, cutting down your meat consumption, reducing your stress level and supplementing your diet with appropriate nutritional supplements will supercharge your immune system and keep viruses, bacteria and parasites at bay. You will also be reducing the number of physician visits and prescriptions you need to endure.

Try to adopt the immune-enhancing diet contained in this chapter along with the ten super-immune-boosting nutrients discussed in chapter 3, and take a daily dose of Sterinol, for at least one month. You will be amazed at the results. You will feel more vibrant and energetic, and colds, flu, aches and pains will be diminished.

THE MIND AND
THE IMMUNE SYSTEM

He who has health has hope; and he who has hope has everything.

—Arabian proverb

It has been almost two decades since the late Norman Cousins published his inspiring story of recovery from disease in *Anatomy of an Illness*. His book broke new ground in describing the potential of the mind to heal the body. It also emphasized the power available when an alliance is formed between physician and patient. *Anatomy of an Illness* sparked a revolution by popularizing the mind/body connection.

His story began in 1964 at a conference abroad, where round-the-clock, high-pressure work produced a state of exhaustion in Cousins. At the same time, he was exposed to excessive hydrocarbons from diesel and jet exhaust. On his trip back to the United States, he became very ill. Within a week he was hospitalized. Tests soon led to the diagnosis of a crippling collagen disease—ankylosing spondylitis. Further tests confirmed that the connective tissue in his spine was disintegrating. One of his doctors told him that he had only a 1 in 500 chance of full recovery. With these odds he decided he had better be more than a passive observer in his treatment.

Cousins's experience in hospital was not unusual. He was subjected to a battery of tests in which four separate blood samples were drawn for four different departments of the hospital on the same day, when one sample would have sufficed. Hospital routine took precedence over the patient's need for rest. X rays, tranquilizers and pain relievers were excessively and indiscriminately offered to him. Above all, the poor-quality hospital food caused him to become malnourished. The experience led to Cousins's fast-growing conviction that a hospital is no place for a person who is seriously ill. For Cousins, the dark side of medicine has given us a world where "the rate at which we die can be exquisitely calibrated." Cousins was fortunate to have a physician who supported his conviction to heal himself and who also had an open mind to alternative treatments.

Familiar with Hans Selye's classic *The Stress of Life*, Cousins reasoned that if negative emotions have negative effects, positive emotions must have positive effects. Deciding to test his hypothesis, he left the hospital and moved into a hotel room staffed with medical attendants. His megadoses of aspirin were replaced with intravenous vitamin C therapy at 25 grams per day. He also discovered the pain-relieving and soporific (sleep-inducing) effects of deep belly laughter. Cousins believed laughter was his best medicine. Soon he became well enough to return to his position as full-time editor at the *Saturday Review*.

Cousins was not the only one to make a connection between the mind and healing. The premise that there might be some connection between physical illnesses and the mind was first postulated in "modern" European thought by William Falconer in 1796. His ideas, presented in a book entitled *The Influence of the Passions Upon Disorders of the Body*, were looked upon with disdain by his colleagues. It took almost two centuries before science again paid any attention to his theory.

THE POWER OF SUGGESTION

Since those days, a great deal more investigation has delved into the mind/body connection. A study conducted at UCLA asked actors to think about certain scenarios where anger, fear and sadness would be exhibited. While they were doing this, samples of their blood were drawn and tested. Researchers found that certain hormones had been released, indicating an effect on the immune system caused by what the actors were feeling. Another study reported in *Science News* asked subjects to perform similar emotion-based tasks. So powerful were these emotional states that finger temperatures soared when the person showed an angry face. Even the thought of pain or watching another's pain induced the body's natural painkilling chemicals. If just thinking about something without a stimulus can produce a physiological response, imagine what happens when you feel extreme stress or loneliness, or have found out you have a serious illness.

A NEW FIELD OF SCIENCE IS BORN

Psychoneuroimmunology is the field of medicine that developed from the findings that emotions and attitudes play a role in how the immune system operates. Other research has followed as the field has expanded to provide evidence that the immune system is hardwired into our nervous system. Researchers such as Candice Pert, Rutgers University, focused on neuropeptides as the biochemical units of emotions. These molecular messengers of cells link the nervous, immune and endocrine systems and are profoundly affected by emotions. Pert's work provided the starting point for numerous scientific investigations that would follow.

Dr. David Felten of the University of Rochester School of Medicine, Rochester, New York, was the first to notice nerve fibers in the middle of vast fields of immune cells. Incredulous, he and his associates looked at each area where immune cells congregate: the spleen and other organs of the immune system. What they found were nerve fibers forming a direct contact with the cells of the immune system. In those early days, it was thought that the immune system functioned autonomously. Now Felten's team had physical evidence to the contrary, that the immune system was hardwired into a communication system with the nervous system, the spleen, lymph nodes and more. Further research found that immune cells also had receptors for the neurochemicals adrenaline and noradrendaline, substances involved in fight-or-flight reactions These findings provided a direct link between the immune system and the mind. The implications of this information were overwhelming: emotions, thoughts and attitudes could have an effect on immune system function in disease development and recovery.

FEELINGS HAVE HEALTH IMPLICATIONS

Researchers have since studied how the immune system responds in people who "feel" lonely, and in those who "feel" they are trapped in a situation. The operative word is "feel." These people may not actually be trapped or alone, but they *feel* they are. In these states, immune function declines and people are left vulnerable to colds, flu and even more serious disease.

Long-term follow-up studies involving women with breast cancer showed that those who received counseling and peer group support survived, on average, twice as long as those who did not. We also know that cancer patients who become part of support groups for cancer, such as Cancer,

Victors and Friends (see Appendix II for cancer organizations), have better survival rates and experience less depression.

Loneliness is a major factor in immune suppression. Studies in which college students were asked to visit nursing home residents showed that the elderly who received weekly visits were less likely to catch colds than those who were not visited. Loneliness is a predictor of lowered immunity in college students as well as the elderly. Students who feel lonely when they go off to college also experience lower immunity and depression.

Our mental state is so important to the body's ability to heal that no therapy should be started without a thorough examination of our emotional being. Imagine the reaction your immune system has to a diagnosis by your doctor that you have a terminal disease. Dr. David Felten recognized the immune implications of the manner in which doctors provide this type of information. Doctors must understand that the way they deliver information about a patient's outcome has a powerful impact and may affect the patient's ability to fight off the disease. Dr. Felten also believes that the very word "patient" has a passive connotation; he suggests we use the word "person," because it suggests someone who is an active participant in his or her life. Many survivors of terminal illness have told us about the day their doctor told them they were going to die. They are survivors because they refused to accept a passive role. They told their doctors that they were going to fight; they weren't beaten yet. One 72-year-old woman said, "Screw you. I am not ready to die yet."

Many illnesses deepen when a negative diagnosis is given. Patients become trapped in a cycle of fear, depression and panic. In a lecture Cousins gave in Victoria, British Columbia, in 1989, he stated that the tragedy is not death but what dies inside us while we live. He told his audience to defy their doctors' verdicts with blazing determination.

When doctors are positive and offer options for healing, patients' outcomes are much more positive. Even patients' attitudes toward their medication can affect the immune system. For instance, negative opinions about medications is evident in unfavorable readings on an electrocardiograph (ECG). We have reports that natural killer cells proliferate in a positive emotional environment, enhancing the body's ability to fight off disease. This is an important reason to ensure that you have a good outlook on life's challenges.

STRESS-COPING STRATEGIES ARE ESSENTIAL

Stress is an everyday occurrence: the kids need to be taken to swimming lessons; the hot-water tank stopped working; your boss wants that report yesterday; and your modem just died. Too many things to do in a day and not enough time to do them. This is the plague of the nineties. Yet certain individuals seem to thrive on the stresses of life and even seek them out, while others are disabled by them and succumb to depression and illness. Scientists are still trying to find out why one person's stress is another's pleasure. Theories about Type A and B personalities have given some insight into the conundrum, but one certainty is that how we cope with our stressors has a direct effect on the immune system.

When we ask children about their most feared situation at school, they tell us it is having to give an oral report in front of their classmates. So stress-inducing is the anticipation of this event that some children become physically ill the day of the presentation. Adults are also affected by this type of situation, with anxiety-related disorders resulting from their fear. Yet other children and adults enjoy the event and sail through it stress-free. Learning to cope with life's challenges is an important step to maintaining your immune system.

Coping strategies *can* be learned. You can adopt simple techniques. For example, think before you say yes to taking on the next project, organizing a school event or driving the team to an event 50 miles from home. Plan your activities and allow time for yourself. Ask for help when you need it and be thankful when it is offered. If you are truly a workaholic or driven to the point of exhaustion, seek counseling. Any type of addiction, even to work, requires understanding to be overcome. One wonderful woman we knew always wanted to help everyone and be part of every committee, but she eventually burned out her immune system and became seriously ill with rheumatoid arthritis. She just could not say no to anyone or anything. Her physician helped teach her some coping strategies and suggested she start wearing the Nike T-shirt that reads "Just Say No." Her friends, colleagues and family began to understand, and she was able to feel good about just being, instead of always doing.

FIND A SILVER LINING IN EVERY CLOUD

In every group there is at least one person who always looks at the bright side of things, even in the face of disaster. An optimistic outlook on life is one predictor of a healthy immune system. Researchers note that people who have a positive attitude to life have much stronger immunity, get fewer viral infections and have more energy.

In *Healthy Pleasures*, Robert Ornstein maintains that people with a positive outlook have better immune function than their negative counterparts. Research confirmed this fact by comparing the blood of individuals who have a positive disposition with the blood of people who have a negative attitude. Optimists had higher immune-boosting helper T-cell counts in relation to suppressor T-cells, which suggests better disease-fighting status. Ornstein declared that good habits contribute less to healthy vitality than a positive attitude toward life that promotes enjoyment of simple pleasures.

TAKE RESPONSIBILITY FOR YOUR RECOVERY

Dr. Dean Black, another prominent researcher, summed it up well when he said, "The physiology of happiness is also the physiology of health, or a sign, at least, that we are using the body as it was designed to be used—not for shrinking in fear, but for stepping forward with boldness and faith." This statement has never before been so important. Persons with cancer, as well as those with serious chronic illness, must take charge of their health and find a practitioner who is willing to work with them not against them. Even more important, don't wait for disease to hit you. Start your immune-boosting program today and you may never have to experience disease.

As represented above, in the story of Norman Cousins, you must start by taking responsibility for your health or illness, learn everything you can about it and mobilize your body's resources to fight back. Seventy-five percent of illnesses are brought under control without medical intervention, and individuals who get actively involved, emotionally and intellectually, are apt to have a more rapid and direct recovery.

Stress is the main factor that puts the immune system into a state of overload and it must be managed. Techniques that teach people how to manage stress are now standard practice for cancer patients, those recovering from heart disease and those with long-term illnesses. Moreover, a strong community of family, friends and colleagues enhance all biological functions in the body.

DON'T TAKE BREATHING FOR GRANTED

Breathing is something we do and rarely think about unless it becomes restricted. Many people don't realize that breathing is a powerful healing tool. It brings valuable oxygen into the system and eliminates carbon dioxide from it. Most women are such shallow breathers that they are oxygen deficient. As often as you remember, fill your lungs with air deep into your abdomen through your nose. Then slowly exhale from your mouth until your lungs are empty. Repeat this five times in a row several times a day. Not only will this destress you, it will help you feel more refreshed. This exercise is especially important if you are bedridden and cannot exercise. By practicing deep breathing, you are bathing your cells in much-needed oxygen and exercising your lungs.

SIMPLE RELAXATION TECHNIQUES

Learning techniques to relax and calm your overstressed mind helps garner the body's ability to heal itself. Yoga, biofeedback training, hypnosis and meditation will not only help you cope with stress, these practices will also help you to get in touch with yourself.

Yoga

Yoga, one of the oldest systems of medicine, is the integration of physical, mental and spiritual energies. Yoga is based on the premise that if the mind is continually restless and out of sorts, the health of the body will suffer. If the body is sick, the mind will be negatively affected. Consciousness and the physical are interconnected, and yoga can help forge an even stronger bridge between the two.

The connection between breath and the mind is the most basic principle of yoga. Breath and its control can help to improve digestion, aid cardiac function, improve oxygen intake, clear the lymph of toxins, reduce the severity of rheumatoid arthritis pain and enhance immune function. It has been found to reduce the frequency of asthma attacks and help individuals cope with anxiety-related symptoms. Posture, breath control and meditation are the basics of yoga but the practice is much more in-depth.

The most common form of yoga taught in North America is hatha yoga. It focuses on various postures (asanas) and breath control. Ask at your local health food store about yoga teachers or classes in your area. Yoga is a wonderful healing method that can be adopted by people of all ages and by those with varying degrees of physical fitness.

Biofeedback Training

Biofeedback training teaches you how to control and change body functions, heart rate, breathing, body temperature, brain waves, muscle action and blood pressure. By consciously affecting these physical functions, you can improve your overall health and well-being.

During university psychology classes we were exposed to the power of biofeedback. Through machinery that evaluated even minor physiological changes in the body, we were taught how to manipulate our body temperature and heart rate. By continually practicing biofeedback techniques, we could improve the ability of our mind to control body functions.

Biofeedback can be easily performed at home. Start by sitting or lying in a quiet place. Clear your mind of other thoughts and concentrate on sending heat down your arms to your hands and through to the tips of your fingers. Before long you will notice that your hands feel warm to the touch. Consider the power of this technique if you visualize heat being sent to the site of, say, a breast tumor. Cancer cells do not survive well under the influence of heat.

Due to the direct connection between the immune system and the nervous system, biofeedback has been shown to reduce incontinence, back pain, ulcers, irritable bowel syndrome, twitching eyelids, fatigue, cerebral palsy, heart irregularities, insomnia, migraines, and to improve pain control and immune function.

Learning to Relax

In a world that never stops, it is difficult for many of us to even consider the dangerous health effects of not taking a few minutes each day to relax. On countless occasions, we have heard people say, "I try to relax but my

Emotional Healing Boosts the Immune System

- Fight with all your determination. Remember Norman Cousins's mantra: Defy the verdict with blazing determination. People who announce that they will beat their disease have much better survival rates.

- See your body's immune cells attacking invaders. Guided imagery is an effective method of boosting your immune system. Whatever image works for you, picture it. Sharks, Star Trek laser guns, gallant soldiers, super warriors, all destroying any and all foreigners in the body. As we have discussed, the mind possesses such power over the immune system that visualizing a hardworking, well-tuned army may help you defend yourself against invaders.

- Learn to like yourself. Suppressed immunity has also been associated with traumas or a lack of love or neglect during childhood. Low self-esteem is also a factor in a depressed immune system.

- Purge negative emotions such as anger and hatred. This is a must if you want your body to heal itself.

- Get help dealing with grief. The loss of a loved one, a divorce or the loss of a job create a form of grief. Immune suppression is the result of grief that never gets dealt with.

- Carpe diem—seize the day and live it to its fullest. Don't worry so much about tomorrow.

- Seek your spiritual side. This does not have to be a religious side, although those with a strong belief in a higher power generally live at peace and feel protected. Most of us believe in something greater than ourselves, a spiritual power that offers solace and helps us find the quiet place within.

- Believe in yourself. Negative self-talk and continually doubting your abilities will hamper your body's ability to heal.

- Notice the beauty around you. Smell the flowers, watch the sunset and listen to the wind.

- Love your family and friends and be forgiving.

- Be good to yourself. Most of us are our own worst enemies, always focusing on our weaknesses and minimizing our strengths. Wake up each day and tell yourself you are a good and useful person.

- Do the things you have always wanted to do. Learn to water-ski, sing in a choir, write a book, tell stories to your grandchildren, walk, garden. Do whatever makes you happy.

mind just won't quit. The things I have to do keep popping into my thoughts." Relaxation, especially deep relaxation, has powerful immune-boosting power. If you have tried and tried and are unable to relax, hire a meditation teacher or hypnotherapist to teach you self-hypnosis. Practice the breathing techniques suggested above and try to adopt the following visualization practice:

Lie on your bed, shut off the ringer on your phone and put a Do Not Disturb sign on the front door. Now, begin by getting into a comfortable position on the bed, arms at your sides, palms facing up. Breathe in deeply through your nose and out through your mouth at least five times. Become aware of the weight of your body on the bed. Breathe. See in your mind's eye the most beautiful place you have ever been to. Maybe it's a waterfall, or a lakeside, or near the ocean with waves rolling onto the beach. Whatever the scene, think only of it, and breathe. You will start to feel as if you are melting into the bed. Your muscles may jerk slightly as they learn to relax. By now a smile has probably moved across your face and you wish you were back at that wonderful spot. Breathe and relax. If thoughts of the tasks you must perform come into your mind while you are learning to relax, don't be annoyed, acknowledge them and return to the concentration of breathing.

Practice this exercise at least once a day, even if only for 5 to 10 minutes. After a few attempts, you will quickly move into a state of relaxation. Stress-reduction techniques take many forms. Find one that works for you, one that can easily fit into your daily schedule.

Combine the suggestions listed in this chapter with your immune system cure nutrition program and you will be armed with a powerful defense package. The mind and body are one unit, interrelated and highly complex. It will take decades for us to truly understand the intricacies of how the mind affects the body's immunity. Today we know that having a positive attitude, a loving family, friends and effective stress-coping strategies help to boost the immune system. Do not wait another day to implement some positive changes in your life.

What you have learned so far will give you the basis for the immune system cure. The following chapters examine certain disease conditions and discuss the amazing results seen in recent research using sterols and sterolins.

Part B

———

THE IMMUNE SYSTEM AND DISEASE

7

CANCER AND IMMUNITY

If you don't take care of your body where are you going to live?

—Lendon Smith, MD

No other medical diagnosis strikes as much fear in the hearts of people as "Cancer." It is a disease that has affected most of us either directly or indirectly, through relatives or friends. Pain, suffering and loss are the connotations this simple word provokes. Fear of the disease is so great that many people avoid visiting the doctor for a diagnosis until their symptoms are unbearable. Most people falsely believe that if they live long enough, they will probably get cancer, and that this diagnosis is an automatic death sentence.

Statistics indicate that one in four people will contract cancer, and one in nine women will be diagnosed with cancer of the breast. Despite heroic measures and enormous amounts of money spent on research, mainstream medicine still has not found a cure, and death rates have been steadily climbing. More than 3 million North Americans have cancer today and another 1.7 million will be diagnosed in 1999. In *Beating Cancer with Nutrition*, Patrick Quillan states that 50 percent of all cancer victims will be alive five years from now, but of the other 50 percent, 40 percent will die of malnutrition, not of cancer. This is an astounding fact. North America is known for its technological advancements, yet people are dying of malnutrition in a country where food is abundant. How can this be?

Survival rates for cancer of the liver, lung, pancreas, bone, and prostate have not improved over the last three decades with conventional cancer treatment. Radiation, chemotherapy and surgery are the current therapies to treat cancer. They cause side effects that are often worse than the cancer itself: extreme nausea and vomiting, hair loss, fatigue, depression, damage to the kidneys and heart, and sometimes other cancers develop later in life as a result of treatment.

NUTRITION: CANCER'S FORMIDABLE FOE

It is possible to live a long and healthy life without living in fear of cancer. Prevention of disease should be the focus. The immune system cure is not a cure for a specific disease; it is a cure for the immune system so that it can function optimally once more to fight off disease, especially cancer, with swiftness and accuracy. The best scenario, of course, is never to get cancer in the first place. A poor diet is believed to be the main cause of the malfunctioning immune system that accounts for 40 to 70 percent of all cancers. How do I protect myself against cancer? you ask. Take this four-step approach:

1. Get your diet on track;
2. Add the nutrients you are missing (chapter 3);
3. Boost your immune system and start eating powerful phytonutrients. Years of research studies now confirm what many doctors knew years ago: plants provide strong medicine (chapter 4); and
4. Ensure that you are happy and fulfilled by exercising and laughing at life's challenges (chapters 6 and 12).

WHY DO WE GET CANCER?

Poor diet, environmental toxins, lack of antioxidants in the diet, chronic stress and feelings of hopelessness are some of the conditions that allow cancers to grow. Although genetics or a family history often predispose an individual to cancer, it can be factored out if super nutrition is adopted. Regardless of your genetic makeup, if you keep your toxic load under control and boost your immunity with optimal nutrition, you can avoid cancer. It is not true that just because you are aging it is inevitable that you will contract cancer. Harness the power of your immune system and cancer will not be a threat.

Viruses are also thought to be a factor in the risk of getting certain cancers: *helicobacter pylori* has been implicated in stomach cancer; human T-cell lymphoma virus has been connected to T-cell lymphoma; human papillomaviruses are thought to be involved in cervical cancer; and the hepatitis virus is linked to liver cancer. A healthy immune system will deal with viruses in a vicious way. Yet these viruses were able to circumvent the body's defenses and cause serious cancers to develop. How?

If you have not been providing your body with antioxidant- and phytonutrient-rich foods, your immune system will be sluggish, making it difficult for your body to detoxify the many substances such as lead, car exhaust, estrogen mimickers (chemicals found in plastics and other substances that mimic estrogen), benzenes, hormones, pesticides, and so on, that it comes in contact with on a daily basis. When this happens, you end up with an unacceptable toxic load or an internal environment that is ready to accept disease. The immune system is confronted with a host of invaders and potential cancer cells every second of the day and, when it is functioning optimally, it skillfully handles each challenge without failing us. Only when the immune system has exhausted its reserves do we become sick.

The liver is the most powerful organ of the body's defense system, not because it fights off invaders, but because it is the organ of the body's detoxification system. If the liver fails, the body experiences such profound toxicity that if the liver is not repaired, death ensues. Hundreds of thousands of chemicals foreign to the body—xenobiotics—are disarmed and disposed of via the liver. This major organ is our speedy toxic disposal system and the immune system would be lost without it. Milk thistle helps support the many functions of the liver. Take 175 mg, three times daily with meals. Look for a supplement that has a standardized extract of silymarin, of at least 80 percent.

WHY ARE NORTH AMERICAN CANCER RATES SO HIGH?

In other parts of the world where nicotine and alcohol consumption are much higher, populations still have significantly lower cancers rates. Japanese citizens smoke twice as much as North Americans and yet their lung cancer rates are 50 percent lower than the North American rate. Their breast cancer rates are 60 percent lower, and prostate cancer is very rare. The French drink more alcohol than North Americans do, and yet they have lower rates of cancers in general. What makes these nations more protected from cancer than North Americans? Diet! Japanese consume more soy, sea vegetables and green tea, all high in phytonutrients, especially the super protectors sterols and sterolins. The wine that the French drink is rich in plant protectors as well.

WHAT IS CANCER?

Normal, healthy cells go through a series of steps to ensure life. They grow, divide and create new cells in a kind of carefully performed, predetermined symphony. During this highly complex reproductive process, the cell's genetic code or DNA is duplicated and transferred to new cells. Normally, this process takes place without error; every once in a while, however, approximately one in a thousand divisions, a mistake occurs. Most mistakes are quickly and correctly repaired, but on occasion a mistake may miss detection and cells will be allowed to perform differently than they were intended.

Cancer begins from normal cells that become renegade cells. These abnormal cells turn the immune system against itself, multiply unchecked, steal nutrients and reroute blood supplies away from normal body functions. Because these turncoat cells are similar to other healthy cells, the immune system often fails to detect and kill them. If the body's defense system is not functioning optimally, the immune system can also miss these marauding cells.

Normal cell conduct organizes cells into their correct location, turns growth off and on as required and ensures that cells do not crowd each other. As a result, normal cells do not travel to parts of the body where they do not belong, and they do not form abnormal structures such as tumors. Cancerous cells, on the other hand, do not follow any hard-and-fast rules; they mutate as often as possible to avoid detection and survive at all cost, even if they kill their host.

The immune system's inability to recognize cancerous cells is believed to be due to our natural killer cell function being depressed. When this surveillance system is malfunctioning, antigens can establish themselves (see chapter 2) and wreak havoc in the body. Tumor cells have not been found to have surface antigens that are any different from normal cells. Without a method of recognizing cancer cells as foreign, the immune system cannot deal with them.

Some cancer cells reproduce at a much faster pace than normal healthy cells. By reproducing at such an increased rate, these cells take over in a certain area and crowd out other cells, often interfering with normal organ or tissue processes. Growths can be either benign or malignant (cancerous). Benign growths are those in which cells divide at an abnormal pace but do not cause damage to the body; for example, fibrocystic breast disease or ovarian cysts. When the abnormal cell growth starts to damage the body, it is then considered cancerous and dangerous to health. Cancerous cells would not be so devastating if they would just stay put, but these cells often break away and travel to other sites in the body, a process called metastasis.

The word "cancer" is derived from the Greek word *karkinos*, which means crab. This word was chosen because of the clawlike appearance of certain tumors. Cancer occurs in most animal species, including birds and fish. Sharks do not get cancer, and much research has gone into finding out why. Cancer can develop in any tissue of the body and it is thought that a cell's DNA may become damaged by any one of the following: radiation exposure, ultraviolet damage from the sun, free radicals, chemical toxins, viruses, hormones, tobacco and alcohol. Each of the above potential DNA-damaging substances can be neutralized with specific nutritional treatments.

Cancer is a complicated disease. Each type of cancer has different traits. Some are slow-growing and easy to treat; others are aggressive and require much more diverse treatment. Drugs that work for one cancer may not have any effect on another. Similarly, each person has unique biochemistry and this must be factored in when treating a person.

ATTITUDE IS THE KEY TO SURVIVAL

Patients who adopt the fighter attitude and refuse to die have higher survival rates than patients who accept the disease and do not play an active role in their treatment. Understanding your cancer is so important to recovery. Educate yourself about conventional treatments and their pros and cons, as well as wholistic therapies. Take an active part in your treatment and stick by your choices.

Continually we hear from patients who have undergone surgery, chemotherapy, radiation and several other therapies in their efforts to combat their disease. They tell us they have tried "everything" and nothing has worked. After evaluating this statement, we usually find that they did try many treatments, but for short periods of time and not in combination with one another. We are not recommending a single cure for cancer; we are suggesting that you adopt the super immune diet that is rich in phytonutrients, combine nutritional supplements, get fresh air and sunshine, be happy and, most important, take Sterinol. If you have cancer, combine these recommendations and stick with them for a minimum of 30 days, the longer the better. None of our suggestions will interact with standard drug therapies and you will be amazed at how well you feel in a short time. You will feel so well, we hope that you adopt this approach to healthy living permanently.

NATURAL THERAPIES PACK A PUNCH

Nature offers us her powerful disease-fighting tools. All we have to do is recognize and use them. Cancer and other diseases of a malfunctioning immune system can easily be avoided and treatment can be amplified if you have started practicing the steps of the immune system cure.

Several fruits and vegetables are especially rich in cancer-blocking agents. Broccoli, cabbage, tomatoes, brussels sprouts, turnips and mustard greens are a few of the most potent cancer fighters. Citrus fruits are rich in D-limonene, another powerful anticarcinogenic that stops toxic agents from damaging the cell's DNA. (See chapters 3, 4 and 5 for more detailed information.)

Ginseng Boosts the Body's Defenses

No cancer treatment or prevention program would be complete without the addition of *Panax ginseng*. Ginseng, rich in saponins, is an adaptogen, a substance which helps the body to find and maintain homeostasis (balance).

Research supporting the cancer-protective effects of ginseng has been astounding. Two long-term studies performed by T. K. Yun in Korea found ginseng to be a potent anticancer agent. In his first study, Yun compared 4,634 people over a period of five years. He found those who consumed ginseng had a 50 percent lower rate of cancers than those who did not take ginseng. In a follow-up study on 1,987 people, Yun found that those taking ginseng for only one year had a 36 percent lower incidence of cancer than non-consumers; and for people who had been taking ginseng for 5 years or longer, he noted a 69 percent lower incidence of cancer.

Ginseng works to protect the body against cancer of the ovaries, larynx, esophagus, pancreas and stomach. It also has a high sterol and sterolin content which, as discussed earlier, has been shown to have a powerful immune-enhancing effect. One capsule of *Panax ginseng* twice daily provides a protective effect.

Marvelous Mushroom Extracts

Mushrooms, including shiitake and maitake, are highly potent anticancer foods that have been used medicinally in Asia for thousands of years. Maitake mushroom, rich in a polysaccharide beta-glucan, possesses powerful immune-enhancing actions and stops or eliminates tumor growth. Researchers at the National Cancer Institute have found that the maitake extract is also effective against the activity of the AIDS virus; they discovered that it stopped the virus from killing T-cells. Supplements containing maitake are available. Take two capsules morning and evening, apart from meals.

A new anticancer drug called Lentinan has been developed in Japan from the shiitake mushroom. So far, Lentinan has been shown to boost interleukin-2 levels and increase the seek-and-destroy activity of macrophages. Shiitake mushrooms also grace our supermarket shelves. This is a wonderful rich-tasting mushroom that when prepared with olive oil and garlic is delicious. For those who dislike eating mushrooms, shiitake extracts are available in capsule form. We recommend 600 mg twice daily.

Wholistic treatments seek to support the body's innate healing abilities while reducing the severity of symptoms that are not only a result of the cancer invading the body, but also of the traditional cancer therapies offered by mainstream medicine. It is known that cancer therapies have many serious side effects including nausea, vomiting, hair loss, painful mouth sores, colds, flu and herpes outbreaks. Patients continually report that they felt worse from conventional treatment than from their cancer. The following research shows that not only can we treat the cancer, we can also reduce the symptoms caused by chemotherapy and radiation.

Sterols and Sterolins: Star Cancer Protectives

Since the mid-1900s, sterols and sterolins have been investigated for their anticancer properties. Over the last nine years, Professor Patrick Bouic and his team at the University of Stellenbosch, Cape Town, South Africa, have been investigating plant sterols and sterolins and their activities on the immune system. They have shown that both beta-sitosterol and its glucoside, beta-sitosterolin, have potent immune properties by activating macrophages to enhance their ability to kill tumors. These natural plant sterols are able to enhance the proliferation of T-cells, and in so doing, enhance the secretion of the cytokines interleukin-2 and gamma-interferon, both immune system regulators. Sterols and sterolins also enhance natural killer cell activity while lowering the pro-inflammatory agent interleukin-6 and the tumor necrosis factor TNF-alpha.

In certain cancers, the secretion of the cytokines interleukin-2 and gamma-interferon, both required for the activation of killer cells, the first line of defense against cancer cells, is defective. In order for the killer cells of the immune system to recognize and destroy tumors, gamma-interferon and interleukin-2 must be present. If these factors are defective, immune cells are not able to recognize and destroy tumor cells, allowing them to develop and damage the body. Sterols and sterolins increase interleukin-2 and gamma-interferon and thereby increase killer cell activity. Sterols and sterolins not only enhance the activity of natural killer cells but also cytotoxic T-cells as well. Remember that cytotoxic T-cells inject killing agents into infected cells to destroy them.

TNF-alpha is another major cytokine that is produced by macrophage cells. In general, its effects cause inflammation (it is pro-inflammatory). TNF-alpha appears to have been designed to recruit immune cells into the site of microbial infections and tissue damage and to prime these cells to act on any offending invader or marauding cancer cell. However, if the immune system is overstimulated due to stress or a heavy toxic load, excessive production of this powerful cytokine can also have undesirable effects, in the form of autoimmune disorders (see chapter 9). TNF-alpha is found to be in excess in certain diseases such as cancer, HIV and autoimmune disorders. Sterols and sterolins effectively reduce TNF-alpha to appropriate levels and interleukin-6 to normal immune-functioning levels.

Research involving HIV patients shows that seven out of ten patients receiving the Sterinol combination had a 64 percent reduction of interleukin-6 after four months of treatment. Although not statistically significant, these results should not be ignored. As mentioned above, Sterinol, a combination of plant sterols, is a powerful immune modulator capable of increasing natural killer cell activity.

Cancer patients undergoing chemotherapy and radiation treatments have noticed a reduction in the associated side effects, nausea, vomiting, hair loss and mouth sores while they were taking Sterinol, 6 capsules daily in divided doses on an empty stomach. To increase absorption, Sterinol should be taken on an empty stomach in the absence of animal fats. Animal fats partially inhibit absorption of sterols and sterolins.

Anti-Tumor Activity of Sterinol

Animal research performed by R. F. Raicht and his colleagues found that when a combination of sterols and sterolins were fed to rats, colon tumors were reduced by 70 percent. In the control group, tumors occurred in 54 percent of the subjects. Sterols and sterolins significantly decreased the proportion of tumor-bearing animals. Although the total number of colon tumors was dramatically reduced, the number of invasive carcinomas was similar in both groups. Beta-sitosterol and beta-sitosterolin may prevent tumors from forming but may not affect the transition of tumors to invasive carcinomas. Sterols and sterolins are easily supplemented through the use of Sterinol in conjunction with a diet including 7 to 10 half-cup servings of fruits, vegetables, seeds and nuts each day.

Dietary factors are thought to be responsible for the large majority of large bowel cancers; studies demonstrating geographic variation in the incidence of colon cancer and changing patterns of disease among migrant populations support this etiology. Researchers now believe strongly that foods contain protective components, especially fruits and vegetables with a high fiber content. In the United States, the vegetarian diets consumed by Seventh-Day Adventists has been credited with lowering the incidence of colon cancer among them. Vegetarian diets are rich in sterols and sterolins and vegetarians have high concentrations of protective sterols in their stool.

Cancer Protection with DHEA and Sterinol

The immune-enhancing link between Sterinol complex and the natural steroid DHEA are now being confirmed. Scientists have shown that DHEA has important immune regulatory actions (see chapter 3) as it increases the secretion of interleukin-2 and gamma-interferon while inhibiting the secretion of interleukin-6 and tumor necrosis factor. Sterinol acts in a similar manner.

When you are under stress, your body releases a hormone called cortisol, which causes cancer-protective DHEA levels to drop. While this is occurring, natural killer cell activity is reduced and the immune system pumps out more interleukin-6, which is an inflammatory factor. These factors combined lead to a dysfunctional immune system that is left vulnerable to attack. Body levels of DHEA normally decline with age, resulting in age-related diseases including cancer, benign prostatic hypertrophy (see chapter 8), arthritis and osteoporosis. Research shows that when aged mice were fed DHEA, their serum interleukin-6 levels declined. It is believed that the Sterinol combination mimics the activities of DHEA with respect to the production of cytokines.

In Canada, DHEA is illegal for sale as it is incorrectly classified under the narcotics act. Sterinol is a safe, effective precursor to DHEA without the side effects (facial hair growth in women and acne) associated with DHEA supplementation.

Sterinol is such a powerful immune modulator, all cancer patients should include it in their cancer treatment program. Sterinol does not have any known drug interactions with current conventional cancer therapies; neither have safety studies on Sterinol shown any side effects from the product. It has also been shown to enhance the activity of interferon cancer treatments. Sterinol is safe, affordable and extremely effective at boosting the immune system. We believe it to be a super-immune supplement. To date, nothing compares to it.

CASE HISTORY

ANTOINETTE TIMMS

Dear Mr. Liebenburg,

Had it been possible for me to convey my thanks in tangible form, I would still not have known how because the gratitude I have in my heart far exceeds expression in material terms.

I am grateful that I could regularly obtain the medication despite the fact that it only recently became available on the market. In my heart of hearts I believe that I would not be alive today had it not been for the mercy from above and your medication.

I have been a puzzle to my orthopedic surgeon, because according to medical research the prognosis is only one year for the type of cancer I had — liposarcoma. I was a receptionist for Professor Lindeque and I witnessed patients dying from this cancer.

This is my seventh year since being operated on for my cancer. Whenever the opportunity presents itself, your product is discussed and consequently, my family and friends are enthusiastic users.

Once more a thousand times thank you for the opportunity offered me to have access to this wonderful medication. I will remain eternally grateful to you.

Antoinette Timms

Cancer Protection Tips

- Avoid bad fats (see chapter 5), eliminate all hydrogenated and partially hydrogenated fats. Eliminate red meat from your diet. Bad-fat diets are associated with colorectal, breast and prostate cancer. Add the healing fats olive and flaxseed oil.

- Enjoy the sun but be aware that our ability to burn is a protection mechanism. It means that we need to seek shade or cover up. Sunlight provides healing benefits, but in short doses and never at midday when the sun is at its hottest between 10 a.m. and 2 p.m; protect your children from sunburn. One serious sunburn involving blistering of the skin dramatically increases the risk of melanoma, a virulent form of skin cancer.

- Choose organic fruits and vegetables and avoid a toxic load of herbicides and pesticides as well as heavy metals. Buy free-range poultry raised without antibiotics and hormone therapy.

- Eat at least 7 to 10 servings of fruits, vegetables, seeds and nuts daily. They are rich in phytonutrients, especially sterols and sterolins.

- Add the ten super immune-boosting nutrients (see chapter 3).

- Ensure that you include in your regimen a daily dose of Sterinol, the most powerful immune modulator known to date.

- Supplement your diet with shiitake and maitake mushroom extracts.

- Quit smoking. If you haven't started to smoke, don't.

- Take milk thistle extract for a healthy liver.

DETOXIFICATION DIET: JUMP-START IMMUNITY

If you have cancer, follow the detoxification diet recommended below for two weeks and then adopt the nutritional recommendations outlined in chapter 5. You will find that these suggestions are a simple, effective way to jump-start your immune system to rid your body of cancer.

Cancer Detoxification Diet

CLASS	FOODS TO INCLUDE	FOODS TO AVOID
Beverages	herb teas, soy, sesame or nut milk, cereal coffee and dandelion coffee	alcohol, cocoa, coffee, milk, soft drinks
Bread	millet, rye, buckwheat, whole wheat bran, corn, seven grain, soya, corn tortillas; only whole grains freshly ground or sprouted, preservative free	bread made with enriched white flour
Cereals	millet, oatmeal, brown and wild rice, barley, cornmeal, seven grain; freshly ground only	processed cereals, flaked, puffed
Dairy	yogurt (unsweetened), tofu soy cheese	cheese
Dessert	fresh whole fruits	canned or frozen fruits, all pastries, Jell-O, custards, ice cream, candy, cakes, cookies
Eggs	none	forbidden in any form

CLASS	FOODS TO INCLUDE	FOODS TO AVOID
Fat	cold-pressed flax, olive, Brazil nut, sesame, sunflower, soy lecithin spread, avocados	butter, shortening, margarine, cottonseed oil, hydrogenated or partly hydrogenated fats, rancid or heated oils
Fish	fresh-water and sea fish; broiled, poached or baked	smoked or salted fish; no shellfish or farm-raised fish
Fruits	organically grown: guava, bananas, cherries, grapes with seeds, nectarines watermelon, berries, apricots, apples, pears, plums, persimmons, peaches, prunes	sprayed, sulphured, canned or frozen
Juices	only fresh unsweetened juices; select from the following: apple and carrot with young beet leaves, chicory, escarole, Swiss chard, watercress, celery	all canned and frozen juices, orange juice
Meat	no meat	beef, pork, bacon, tongue; smoked, salted or processed; cold cuts, hot dogs
Poultry	free-range, maximum of twice per week; take with digestive enzymes	
Milk	kefir, sesame or nut milks, soy milk, yogurt	all non-fermented dairy

CLASS	FOODS TO INCLUDE	FOODS TO AVOID
Nuts	limited amounts of all fresh, raw-in-the-shell nuts, particularly Brazil nuts and almonds; raw nut butters made fresh in blender; choose nuts from list of sterols and sterolins in chapter 4	roasted or salted nuts and peanuts
Potatoes	baked or steamed with jackets	French fries, chips, grilled
Vegetables	all vegetables organically grown, steamed	frozen or canned, sprayed
Salads	organically grown salad greens, shredded carrots, apple, celery, etc.	iceberg lettuce
Dressings	only made with organic cold-pressed oils, with apple-cider vinegar and recommended seasonings	
Seasonings	chives, garlic, parsley, sage, thyme, kelp, vegetable and herb seasonings	black pepper and table salt; sodium chloride or mono-sodium glutamate (MSG)
Seeds	sunflower, pumpkin, chia, inside the pits of apricots	roasted or salted
Sprouts	any seed sprouted at home; store sprouts may be contaminated	potato sprouts poisonous
Sugars	in moderation: raw honey, maple syrup	white or brown sugar; all sugar substitutes
Soups	plenty of homemade with vegetable stock, miso	canned, creamed, bouillon, consommé and beef stock

---

PROTECT YOUR PROSTATE

In time we hate that which we often fear.

—William Shakespeare

Few men ever consider their prostate gland until it starts to give them problems. According to a report in *Vitamin Research News*, a 1995 survey published in the *London Times* found that 89 percent of the men surveyed did not know where the prostate is located. Considering the grim statistics that most men over the age of 40 will experience some type of prostate problem that will affect their sexual and urinary function, it is an important gland to understand if we want to prevent disease.

Small in size but grand in problems this gland accounts for a staggering 2.7 million doctor visits in North America each year. The prostate gland has tremendous influence over the ability to perform sexually as well as to urinate. The location of this gland is the cause of most of its problems. The small, chestnut-size gland is located just below the bladder and is wrapped around the urethra. The urethra is the pathway for sperm and urine, and if the prostate gland begins to swell, it will alter normal urinary flow and the ejaculation of sperm.

At orgasm, the critical point of sexual stimulation, the muscles surrounding the prostate and the bladder squeeze semen and other seminal fluids from the prostate, testes and seminal sacs into the urethra and out through the penis. When the prostate gland swells due to infection, inflammation or other causes, the prostate can fail to produce the fluids

Prostate Problems

EARLY WARNING SIGNS

- an increased number of visits to the bathroom along with a frequent sensation of needing to urinate, especially at night
- a reduction in the force and caliber of urination
- a burning sensation during urination
- chronic constipation
- trouble starting or stopping a urine stream
- painful ejaculation
- infertility

MORE SERIOUS SYMPTOMS*

- constant pain or stiffness in the pelvis, hips, upper thighs or lower back
- loss of weight, exhaustion, nausea or vomiting
- blood in urine or semen

***If you have any of these symptoms, seek medical diagnosis and treatment immediately.**

required for reproduction, and infertility may result. Painful ejaculation is also the result of prostate swelling.

As mentioned above, urinary dysfunction also occurs as a result of a swollen prostate gland. Men with this problem often experience a continual urge to urinate, yet no urination ensues. Moreover, a reduction in the force of urination may result in the bladder failing to empty fully and infection may result. A burning sensation or pain upon urinating often accompanies this disorder. These symptoms can become gradually worse if the reason for the prostate swelling is not determined and treated.

SIMPLE TEST TO PROTECT YOUR SEX LIFE

Men often fail to seek diagnosis and treatment for the above symptoms because they want to avoid a prostate examination or fear a cancer diagnosis.

Many men have heard so many horror stories about prostate treatments causing impotence that they are afraid to seek help. Moreover, prostate problems are not a common topic of conversation among men, since it is perceived to be a private problem. With prostate cancer now the second leading cancer killer in men, behind lung cancer, talking about this problem, learning about treatment options and visiting your physician are intelligent steps to take.

Prostate problems can be broken down into three categories: benign prostatic hypertrophy (BPH); an enlarged prostate, prostatitis or inflammation of the prostate; and cancer. Under the umbrella of prostate problems, cancer is the rarest prostate problem. It is the second leading cancer, but BPH and prostatitis are much more common prostate problems.

A prostate exam is a simple procedure that men over the age of 50 should have each year. Women have been trained to visit their physician for an annual Pap smear in order to rule out infection and cancer of the cervix, a test that saves many lives every year. Men need to be trained likewise, to understand the importance of a digital prostate exam. It is a simple procedure that takes less than half a minute. The doctor will ask you to lie on your side on the examining table and fold your knees to your chest, or to stand and bend over the side of the table. The physician will then insert a well-lubricated, gloved finger in the rectum and feel for the prostate. Although not a pleasant experience, these few seconds can mean the health of your sex life and urinary function, so relax—it will be over quickly. A healthy prostate is firm to the touch, smooth and pliant. Hard nodules or lumps and bumps indicate a need for further tests to rule out a more serious condition. An ultrasound scan and/or biopsy (see below) may be performed to confirm any diagnosis.

PSA Test

The prostate specific antigen (PSA) test evaluates a protein that can diagnose prostate cancer at a very early stage before the rectal exam would be able to locate a lump or tumor. The higher the PSA test score, the more likely prostate cancer is present.

There is much controversy regarding the PSA test though. PSA testing misses approximately 33 percent of prostate cancer cases, and on the other hand, it diagnoses cancer 60 percent of the time when none is present.

PSA EXAM VALUE	MEANING OF PSA SCORES
0 – 4	thought to be normal
4 – 10	indicates BPH or prostatitis
10 – 20	may indicate cancer
20 and up	cancer

Unnecessarily, serious anguish is experienced by men who are mistakenly diagnosed with cancer. The National Cancer Institute has stopped recommending the PSA test due to its unreliability, but the Canadian and American Cancer societies are still recommending it. A new, more reliable PSA test will be available in the near future.

Biopsy

Biopsy is normally only performed when a physician has evaluated the earlier screening methods mentioned, especially if an ultrasound shows a potential tumor. Usually a biopsy is performed on an outpatient basis at the hospital. A local anesthetic is administered and many prostate samples are gathered. Biopsies help determine if a tumor is slow-growing, malignant (cancerous) or benign, or if it is an aggressive type. Results will help determine the type of treatment therapy to be used.

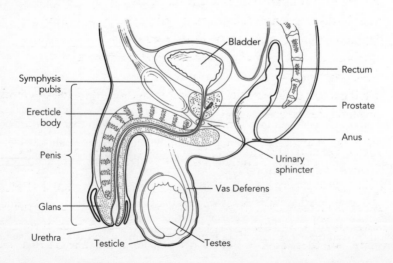

The purpose of this chapter is not to look at prostate cancer or prostatitis, which is generally the result of a bacterial infection, but to provide safe, natural remedies for benign prostatic hyperplasia, the most common and stubborn prostate problem and its prevention.

BENIGN PROSTATIC HYPERTROPHY (BPH)

If your days and nights start revolving around trips to the bathroom, a problem with your prostate is brewing. Men frequently complain that they are exhausted from having to rise 4 to 6 times each night to urinate. What is even more frustrating is that half the time, urination won't begin, and when it starts, the urine just dribbles out. These are some of the first signs of benign prostatic hypertrophy (BPH), an enlargement of the prostate which interferes with normal sexual function and urinary flow.

Less talked about than cancer but very prevalent and extremely aggravating, BPH affects more than 25 million men in North America. Some myths that must be dismissed include: BPH is not cancer; does not turn into cancer; and does not increase the risk of developing prostate cancer. Symptoms of BPH may or may not be present in cases of cancer. The symptoms listed in the more serious section on page 114 are directed to the possibility of prostate cancer.

BPH may present only one symptom or many. These include:

- an impaired urine stream that is less forceful than it used to be
- having to wait until your urine stream begins
- your bladder no longer fully empties and you have to visit the bathroom minutes after you have just been there
- dribbling of urine long after you have stopped urinating
- urinating every hour
- having to get up several times at night even though you did not drink any fluids before going to bed

One cause of BPH is related to the hormone testosterone, produced by the testes and the adrenal glands. As a man ages, his conversion of testosterone to the active form of testosterone, dihydrotestosterone (DHT), increases. With more DHT the tissues of the prostate grow faster and the old tissues are not removed fast enough; a buildup of tissue results in an enlarged prostate. Another cause of BPH may be chronic constipation that puts

Going Toward the Light

BPH is such a common problem that even birthday cards use it as a subject:

On his birthday, an old guy visits his physician for his annual exam. The guy says to his doctor, "I feel great but I have these weird spiritual experiences." The doctor says, "What do you mean?" The old guy says, "When I get up in the middle of the night to use the bathroom, I open the door and a light turns on for me. When I'm finished, the light turns off. The doctor says, "I've seen this before in guys your age. You are not having a spiritual experience. You're peeing in the refrigerator."

added pressure on the prostate by an overly full rectum. These factors may play a role, but diet can change the way the body produces and manages its hormones and it can also alleviate constipation.

Contrary to popular opinion, BPH is not inevitable. Although almost every man who lives long enough gets BPH, it does not mean you have to contract the disorder. Diet and lifestyle seem to be the key factors as to whether or not you get BPH. Adopting the super immune diet for as little as 30 days will help heal BPH. Those affected by BPH report that after they eliminated spicy foods, coffee, alcohol, tobacco and sugar, their symptoms very quickly abated. Add the immune-boosting nutrients discussed in chapter 3, with a little extra zinc at 60 mg per day, and you will feel even better.

Plant Sterols for Benign Prostatic Hypertrophy

Plant nutrients are powerful immune boosters. The superstar phytonutrients sterols and sterolins have been researched for more than 20 years in Germany for their effect on benign prostatic hypertrophy. The product used in the studies is Harzol, a combination of sterols and sterolins manufactured by the same company that makes Sterinol. Strict German food and drug controls have prevented updating Harzol to the potency of Sterinol, but even with this product the studies produced excellent results for BPH sufferers.

In one double-blind, placebo-controlled study 200 patients, of an average age 65 and with a diagnosis of BPH, were recruited. After a four-week washout period where medication was restricted, patients were given 20 mg of sterols and 200 mcg of sterolins, three times daily on an empty stomach for six months. In contrast to the placebo group, the sterols and sterolin group showed a decrease in the International Prostate Symptom Score (IPSS) (see chart on page 114) and an increase in peak urinary flow from 9.9 ml per second to 15.2 ml per second, as well as a lower residual urinary volume. There were no side effects reported in this research. Based on the conclusions of this study, sterols and its glucoside sterolin are an effective treatment for BPH.

In a discussion of this work published in the *Quarterly Review of Natural Medicine*, naturopathic physician Ronald Reichert stated that although the authors of the study do not examine the mechanism of action for sterols and sterolins, we can look at how the phytosterols from the herb *Pygeum africanum* operate. Sterols from pygeum seem to inhibit the production of prostaglandins, especially PGE2 and PGF2 alpha, both of which are important mediators in the inflammatory process. A decrease in inflammation lowers local prostate congestion, resulting in fewer symptoms and improved peak urinary flow.

The researchers also contrasted the effectiveness of beta-sitosterol with Proscar, a 5-alpha-reductase inhibitor (see below). They noted that plant sterols increased peak urine flow as well as, if not better than, Proscar, from 9.9 to 15.2 ml per second for beta-sitosterol compared with 9.6 to 10.4 ml per second for Proscar. Long-term safety studies (a safety study is performed to determine if there are any side effects of a medication; long-term studies are performed longer than six months) involving 250,000 persons have found sterols and sterolins to have no side effects. An extremely rare sterol storage disorder called sitosterolemia does exist, but fewer than 28 cases have been reported worldwide.

In Germany, Dr. Klippel has been studying the effects of sterols and sterolins on BPH in double-blind, placebo-controlled studies for almost a decade. He has found that sterols and sterolins reduce inflammation and congestion, reduce edema, normalize estrogen and stop the abnormal proliferation of prostate tissue. The first study that he oversaw was designed according to the guidelines of the International Consultation on BPH, an international organization that developed the list of symptoms and the International Prostate Scoring System. This study required long-term

Research Design

Double-blind, placebo-controlled studies are regarded by researchers as the most valid form of research design.

Double-blind means that neither the patient nor the researcher knows whether any particular patient is getting the test substance or the placebo. Every container of substance and every patient are assigned code numbers that are meaningless to all except the researcher who analyzes the results when the test period is concluded.

A **placebo** is an inactive substance in a form that looks exactly like the substance being tested.

treatment for six months; it needed to be placebo controlled; and it was required to use the International Prostate Treatment Score (IPT) as the main parameter. One hundred and seventy-seven patients were enrolled in 13 study centers across Germany. Because of the encouraging results, it was the first study on BPH to be reported in an international, peer-reviewed journal. Also interesting is that improvements in the IPT Score were seen within 30 days.

Sterols and sterolins should be the basis for any BPH therapy as they are effective, affordable and easy to supplement. Take Sterinol, 1 capsule three times daily on an empty stomach. Tom, an 84-year-old retired engineer living in British Columbia, found that after only 30 days on Sterinol, his nighttime visits to the bathroom were reduced by 50 percent. He was overjoyed at being able to sleep better at night and very encouraged that the therapy was working so quickly. Up until this point, he had tried many natural therapies to get his BPH under control, with no success.

Pumpkinseeds, the herbs *pygeum africanum* and *serenoa repens* (saw palmetto) are also effective in treating and preventing BPH. Interestingly, they also contain sterols and sterolins; *pygeum africanum* in standardized form contains 14 percent beta-sitosterol. We believe that their effectiveness may be due to the sterols and sterolins they contain. The dosage these herbs contain is much less than that of Sterinol and not in the correct ratio to have any immune modulating activity. We recommend that Sterinol be the basis for your BPH program, to which you can add the following remedies if required.

Saw Palmetto (*Serenoa repens*)

Extracts of saw palmetto are being used worldwide to treat BPH. Numerous double-blind, placebo-controlled clinical trials have demonstrated that saw palmetto improves urinary flow, alleviates nocturnal voiding and reduces the number of times one needs to urinate during the day. Saw palmetto extract has been compared to Proscar, a prescription drug prescribed to BPH patients in North America. Results showed that saw palmetto was equivalent or better in its action without the side effects associated with Proscar (impotence, loss of sex drive and abnormal ejaculations) and it was less expensive.

Inside the prostate an enzyme transforms testosterone into a new compound called 5-dihydrotestosterone (DHT). It is believed that DHT stimulates new cells to be deposited in the prostate, and swelling and urine flow to be decreased. Scientists believe that a reduction in this conversion will prevent BPH or at least shrink the prostate to alleviate symptoms. In tests, Proscar prevented the enzyme 5-alpha reductase from converting testosterone to DHT.

Saw palmetto works by blocking the conversion of testosterone to dihydrotestosterone (DHT) by inhibiting 5-alpha reductase and by preventing the binding of DHT. The action of this increases the elimination of DHT. It also reduces the inflammation associated with BPH and reduces the effects of estrogen and progesterone on the prostate.

French researchers discovered that saw palmetto berries are rich in essential fatty acids as well as sterols and sterolins. Sterinol contains a higher percentage of sterols and sterolins than saw palmetto and should be the basis for a BPH treatment program.

Pygeum africanum

Pygeum africanum is a herb used to treat urinary disorders. It is anti-inflammatory, anti-edema and has cholesterol-lowering capabilities. Clinical trials have shown that it reduces BPH symptoms. The herb effectively inhibits the conversion of testosterone and increases blood flow to the prostate.

In a study of 18 patients with BPH or chronic prostatitis, pygeum was found to improve all urinary symptoms within 60 days. In another placebo-controlled clinical trial of 120 patients with BPH, the pygeum group experienced a significant reduction in the number of daily trips to the bathroom and more complete emptying of the bladder.

An international, multicentered, double-blind controlled study involving 236 patients with BPH, over 60 days, showed an improvement again on all urinary symptoms. Dosages of 150 mg of standardized pygeum per day are required.

Tomatoes Protective against BPH

We have already told you about the anti–prostate cancer properties of the phytonutrient found in tomatoes called lycopene. Be sure to add tomatoes to your daily diet. For more information, see chapter 4.

Omega-3 and 6 Oils Reduce BPH Symptoms

Research in the early 1940s confirmed that after several weeks of supplementation with omega-3 alpha-linolenic fatty acids and omega-6 linoleic fatty acids, 12 out of 19 men with BPH had no residual urine left in the bladder after urination. This is a very important fact as infection is often a result of residual urine. Moreover, 13 out of the 19 men studied no longer complained of nighttime wakenings to urinate.

Fatty acids work by decreasing inflammation in the prostate. Essential fatty acids work by promoting hormone-like prostaglandins that prevent excessive prostatic growth by blocking testosterone from binding to the prostate. Essential fatty acids are also excellent anti-inflammatory, antibacterial agents. Take 2 tablespoons of flax oil daily and add 1 tablespoon of pumpkinseed oil. Pumpkinseeds are a good source of zinc, sterols and sterolins and essential fatty acids important in the treatment of BPH.

Cranberry Cures Urinary Problems

Cranberry is one of nature's best weapons against cystitis and urinary tract infections. For years, doctors have been recommending that patients drink cranberry juice to prevent urinary tract infections. At one time, scientists believed that cranberry acidified the urine and in the process killed invading bacteria that could cause infection. However, Dr. Anthony Sabota, a scientist at Youngstown State University, Ohio, offered another explanation. His studies suggest that cranberry prevents bacteria from attaching to the wall of the bladder, thus allowing potential bacteria to be flushed out of the body before they can cause infection. For men with BPH who have problems eliminating urine from the bladder, cranberry may help ward off infections. Choose cranberry juice that does not contain sugar or artificial sweeteners. Remember that sugar reduces the ability of the immune cells to attack invaders. Capsules containing cranberry extracts are also available.

THE RIGHT FATS

We know there is a strong correlation between the incidence of prostate cancer and countries where men eat large amounts of saturated fat from red meat. In contrast, countries like Japan, where the diet is higher in fruits, vegetables, soy and rice, prostate cancer rates are low. It was also found that

Odds of Being Diagnosed with Prostate Cancer	
AGE	ODDS OF DIAGNOSIS
20–39	Insignificant
40–44	1 in 48,640
45–49	1 in 9,085
50–54	1 in 1,943
55–59	1 in 624
60–64	1 in 240
65–69	1 in 122
70–74	1 in 81
75–79	1 in 65
80–84	1 in 58
85 up	1 in 63

Source: American Cancer Society: Number of Men by Age, from the U.S. Bureau of the Census

when Japanese men moved to the United States, a country where red-meat consumption is high, their prostate cancer rates increased. Although there is no connection between BPH and prostate cancer, prostate health in general is affected by the foods we eat, especially fats.

In an article entitled "Lowering Bad Fat Intake Slows Growth of Prostate Cancer," Jack Challem, publisher of the newsletter *Nutrition Reporter*, reported on a Sloan-Kettering experiment in which researchers transplanted human prostate cancers into mice; once the cancers started growing, they divided the mice into several groups. Their diets were the same except for fat intake, which was 40.5, 30.8, 21.2, 11.6 or 40.5 percent fat from corn oil, comparable to the typical American diet. After 11 weeks, the mice that consumed only 21.2 percent fat had tumors roughly half the size of those of the mice consuming the highest-fat diet. The researchers wrote in the *Journal of the National Cancer Institute* that dietary modification of fat resulted in slower tumor growth even after the formation of measurable tumors. They also noted that prostate specific antigen (PSA) levels decreased along with tumor size.

REGULAR SEX IS IMPORTANT TO PROSTATE HEALTH

Regular sexual intercourse is essential to prostate health. Unfortunately, a decline in sexual activity as we age is thought to be normal and may be related to the rise in prostate problems.

Sex is not only good for your prostate but for your mental and emotional health as well. As we learned in chapter 6, a loving relationship is a powerful healing instrument. Immune cells flourish when we feel content and loved. What we are telling you is that sex is good for you.

The congestion that occurs in the prostate when it is not allowed to ejaculate causes inflammation. If this is a continual state of affairs, the prostate suffers and swelling is the result.

9

AUTOIMMUNE DISEASES

Those who do not find time every day for health must sacrifice a lot of time one day for illness.

—Father Sebastion Kneipp

A balanced immune system normally distinguishes friend from foe and only attacks foreign invaders, avoiding the body's own tissues. Occasionally, however, our immune system's weaponry turns against itself, causing destruction and, in severe cases, death. The illnesses that are a result of this return of friendly fire are called autoimmune diseases.

Autoimmune diseases can involve any system in the body, although some organs and tissues appear to be more susceptible than others. Five percent of the adult population in North America is afflicted with one or more autoimmune diseases, and two-thirds of those are women. Autoimmune diseases are usually diagnosed in early adulthood, generally after a bout of illness or severe stress. Remember that stress and illness cause imbalances in the immune system and are causally linked to the diseases of today. People affected by autoimmune disorders often experience periods of remission, during which the symptoms disappear, alternating with periods of acute episodes, during which symptoms flare up. Other people see their symptoms progressively worsen and their condition deteriorate.

Heredity is a factor involved in an individual's predisposition to autoimmune disease, but as is found in studies involving twins, if one twin is diagnosed with an autoimmune disease, the other has a higher risk, but does not necessarily acquire the disease. Many other factors, discussed below, are involved in the immune system's turning upon the body.

WHAT IS AUTOIMMUNITY?

Autoimmune disorders occur when the immune system begins to attack the body. Among the many hypotheses to explain the cause of autoimmunity are: viral or bacterial infection; stress; and genetic susceptibility.

Infection is considered the main culprit as it often precedes the onset of an autoimmune diagnosis. Viruses and bacteria have devised methods to avoid detection thereby allowing themselves access to the body. Certain viruses provide the immune system with strings of amino acids that are so similar to those of the body that they are thought of as "self" until some anomaly tells otherwise (see chapter 2). As a result, the immune system can become confused and think it is attacking an invader, when it is actually attacking itself. One well-known virus, the adenovirus type 2, does just that. It has amino acid sequences that are very similar to that of the myelin proteins that surround the nerves in the body. When the body responds to this common virus, it may also mistakenly attack myelin. This type of response may be critical in the initiation of autoimmune disease. Other infectious organisms implicated in causing immune dysregulation include mycobacterium tuberculosis, chlamydia, salmonella and yersinia. It is proposed that these organisms lead to the production of an autoantigen which makes an autoimmune response ensue.

> An **antigen** is a protein marker on the surface of cells that identifies the cell as self or non-self and stimulates the production of antibodies. Antigens on the body's own cells are called **autoantigens**.

So why is it that everyone who is exposed to a virus does not acquire an autoimmune disease? Many factors have to be in place for the immune system to become disrupted. Genetic makeup and a weakened immune system due to stress, poor diet or exposure to environmental toxins all contribute to whether or not the immune system is compromised.

Autoimmune diseases are often worse in women than men. Scientists believe that the female hormone estrogen may be the reason for this.

The hormone estrogen may interplay with certain immune factors that enhance the action of the inflammatory response, increasing antibodies that attack certain tissues in the body. An over abundance of estrogen or estrogen-dominance may be a factor in the prevalence of autoimmune conditions in women.

Autoimmune Diseases

DISEASE	AFFECTED ZONE
Ankylosing spondylitis	spine
Rheumatoid arthritis	cartilage and joint linings
Multiple sclerosis	brain and spinal cord
Juvenile diabetes	cells that excrete insulin
Systemic lupus erythematosus	DNA, platelets, most tissues
Myasthenia gravis	nerves and muscles
Grave's disease	thyroid function
Crohn's disease & Celiac disease	gut
Insulin-dependent diabetes mellitus	pancreatic beta-cells
Idiopathic thrombocytopenic purpura	platelets
Psoriasis	skin
Pernicious anemia	gastric parietal cells
Autoimmune hemolytic anemia	red blood cell membranes

The above lists only a few of the many autoimmune diseases known today. They all have one common thread—the body turning against itself, thereby causing disease and destruction. Although each autoimmune disease involves different tissues and organs, the process that causes the disease in the first place is the same.

CONVENTIONAL TREATMENTS

Conventional treatment protocols have serious drawbacks. They most often include anti-inflammatory drugs or general immune system suppressants such as corticosteroids and cyclosporine. The side effects from immune suppressors are so severe they are only prescribed for the most serious cases of autoimmunity. Suppressing the immune system leaves you highly susceptible to infections and cancer.

Dangers of Pain Medication

North Americans spend more than 3.9 billion dollars on over-the-counter pain medications. Acetaminophen is the most commonly used painkiller, followed by non-steroidal anti-inflammatories (NSAIDs) such as ibuprofen and aspirin. More pain medications are purchased for the control of arthritis symptoms than for any other disorder.

Safety is an issue. Long-term use of NSAIDs causes 20,000 deaths in the United States annually. Side effects are common: gastrointestinal complaints including bleeding, nausea and vomiting, liver damage, stomach ulcers, allergic reactions, immune system depression, mental confusion and kidney failure. Adverse drug interactions are not uncommon and central nervous system toxicity is at great risk when the medication indomethacin is prescribed. Patients receiving corticosteroids and NSAIDs together are at 15 times greater risk for peptic ulcer disease than those receiving no medications.

One study published in the *New England Journal of Medicine* found that NSAIDs are the cause of 15 percent of all drug-induced cases of kidney failure. The *Lancet* study found that NSAIDs contribute to cartilage destruction. Arthritis causes cartilage destruction, and the very medication needed to control the pain of that destruction causes it. This is a very disturbing idea indeed.

Acetaminophen is not immune from problems either. When taken in higher than recommended doses, it causes liver damage. Acetaminophen overdose is the leading cause of acute liver failure and causes 10 percent of all cases of kidney failure. Combining alcohol with acetaminophen can be fatal.

There are several safe pain-relieving options. These include bromelain, white willow bark and caffeine. Bromelain taken between meals works to inhibit prostaglandin production and reduce inflammation. Doses of 1,500 mg are required to relieve the pain of rheumatoid arthritis (RA). White willow bark naturally contains salicylic acid, the same ingredient found in aspirin. Moreover, in comparison studies, 200 mg of caffeine was more effective than 400 mg of ibuprofen at eliminating the pain of headaches. These natural substances work quickly and without the side effects associated with standard over-the-counter pain relievers.

Castor Oil for Pain Control

Castor oil compresses are an excellent way to alleviate pain. Take several squares of 100 percent cotton flannel. Cut into six pieces the size of the area you want to treat. Pour castor oil onto each flannel piece until it is evenly moist, not dripping. Place each piece one on top of the other on the area in need of pain reflief. Cover with a towel and hot water bottle (not an electric heating pad as they emit harmful energy) until the heat dissipates. Most people experience pain relief quickly. For stubborn pain, use a second application of heat. This treatment works especially well for back, joint and abdominal pain.

IMMUNOLOGICAL WEAPONRY 101

Let's recap how a normal immune response proceeds. A healthy, balanced immune system relies on B-cells to produce antibodies that will destroy invading bacteria, viruses, fungi and parasites before they get a chance to enter the healthy cells of the body. T-cells are the immune cells that control and regulate the immune response or the call to battle. T-cells are divided into two groups, helper T-cells and cytotoxic T-cells. The helper T-cells are then broken down into two further groups called T_H1 helper cells and T_H2 helper cells. These cells have very specific functions and each type releases certain immune factors that help or hinder the immune response as required. When the T_H1 and T_H2 cells are in balance, health is maintained. If an overabundance of one or a deficiency of the other occurs, disease sets in. T_H1 helper cells release interleukin-2 and gamma-interferon. T_H2 releases interleukin-4, 6 and 10, which enhance the ability of B-cells to produce antibodies.

If there is a reduction in the number or activity of T_H1 cells, natural killer cell activity, the first line of defense against invaders, is decreased. When T_H2 is not in balance, an overabundance of antibodies are produced, which cause inflammation.

Many opportunistic invaders such as viruses have devised a mechanism of avoiding detection in the human body by taking up residence inside healthy cells. B-cells are often unable to mount an antibody assault once the invader is hiding in a host cell. The immune system has evolved to deal with most of these types of invaders by harnessing the power of cytotoxic T-cells.

Cytotoxic T-cells are told to become killing machines by T_H1 cells so that they can kill any invader that has been able to get into a healthy cell. In order to get at the disease-causing organism hiding in the cell, cytotoxic T-cells have to kill the host cell as well.

The immune system is finely tuned to adapt to changes that occur either when a virus or bacteria invades or when a cancerous cell is lurking. When the T_H1 arm of the immune defense system is deficient, natural killer cell activity is reduced, infection and disease result, and chronic inflammation and eventually tissue damage as seen in autoimmune diseases is inevitable.

PLANT STEROLS AND STEROLINS RETURN BALANCE

Our bodies are designed to protect us, not harm us. Only in the face of complete confusion will the powerful army we have inside ourselves turn on itself. Stress is the main factor. It causes a host of immune dysfunctions (see chapter 12). Infections caused by viruses and bacteria are another cause of the immune system going awry. Genetics plays a minor role and nutrition plays the leading role in the promotion of immune disharmony.

Plant foods are so full of potent ingredients that food alone can be your best medicine in maintaining immune system health. We know from the research presented in chapter 4 that the powerful ingredients in a simple tomato can protect you from cancer. Seeds and nuts are so rich in healing ingredients, the US Federal Drug Administration (FDA) and Canadian Health Protection Branch (HPB) might just classify them as drugs. Now we are also aware of the superstar power of the plant fats found in all plant-based foods.

Plant sterols and sterolins are so effective at modulating the immune system—that is, putting it back in balance—that one day autoimmune disorders may become history. Sterinol, the combination of plant sterols and sterolins as found in nature, modulate the functions of the body's T-cells by enhancing their ability to divide; therefore, we would have more T-cells to add to the army. They also promote the secretion of interleukin-2 and gamma-interferon. Sterinol does this without enhancing the action of T_H2 helper cells, which are implicated in promoting inflammation and producing more antibodies. This is crucial because autoimmune diseases are caused by the body producing antibodies against itself and the disease is made worse by the severe inflammation that occurs. Both interleukin-2 and gamma-interferon are able to shut off the immune system's antibody-producing machinery.

Let's look at rheumatoid arthritis, for example. It is thought that the overactivity of B-cells is directly involved in the release of antibodies that attach themselves to synovial joint tissue, which then cause destruction. Those antibodies then form complexes with other antibodies within a joint, a process that causes the severe inflammation seen in RA sufferers. At the sites of active tissue destruction, it has been found that there are very high levels of the cytokines: interleukin-6, tumor necrosis factor alpha and interleukin-1—all factors that promote inflammation. Researchers have shown that the destructive process seen in RA can be induced in normal cartilage by adding the fluid from a rheumatoid arthritis patient's synovial fluid to the healthy cartilage.

Patrick Bouic and his research team have shown that Sterinol is beneficial in the control of autoimmune disease. Sterinol modulates the immune response to autoimmunity and controls the disease by preventing the damage caused by the inflammation. More important, however, it is able to reverse the immune abnormality at the site of the disease. The major difference between the use of conventional medicines and Sterinol in the control of autoimmunity is that conventional drugs are mainly aimed at inhibiting the entire immune response and the inflammatory process, hence the use of anti-inflammatory and immune-suppressing drugs. Conventional treatments are also not without side effects and dangers: they leave the person affected open to common and opportunistic infections because the immune system is kept suppressed to protect the body from the onslaught of the immune response. It is important to note that immune-suppressed patients are more prone to the development of life-threatening tumors and carcinomas.

Sterinol is entirely different in its function in that it targets the abnormality and corrects the immune dysfunction. As mentioned above, many factors can lead to the malfunction of the immune response, especially poor nutrition. It therefore stands to reason that many chronic diseases are preventable by ensuring the intake of sterols and sterolins naturally found in plants. Sterinol is a natural, non-toxic substance. It is free of any side effects and will not cause immune suppression. In a clinical trial, 25,000 volunteers took 1 Sterinol capsule, three times daily, over an extended period of time. No side effects were reported.

Sterinol is a revolutionary approach to the treatment of autoimmune disease. Clinical trials are currently under way to confirm the results of preliminary studies on the effects of sterols and sterolins on rheumatoid arthritis, allergies, CIN III cervical lesions, HIV and chronic fatigue syndrome. We are impressed with the positive results seen in patients taking part in the trials. See the end of the chapter for case studies of people who experienced "permanent remission" of their autoimmune symptoms.

If you suffer from any of the autoimmune diseases mentioned in this chapter, we recommend that you take 1 capsule of Sterinol, three times a day, on an empty stomach or an hour before meals. Take 1 capsule upon rising, 1 in the afternoon and 1 before going to bed. Results vary depending on the severity of the autoimmune disease, but those who have been using the product experience significant results within 30 days. If you have insulin dependent diabetes, you will need to monitor your insulin requirements. We have seen patients require less insulin within a matter of weeks.

HEAVY METAL POISONING IS A FACTOR IN AUTOIMMUNITY

Environmental pollution is a serious problem. By the time our children are six months old, they have received 30 percent of their total lifetime toxic load. Poisons from pesticides, herbicides, chemical fertilizers, industrial wastes and automobile exhaust make up the vast percentage of toxins we are exposed to on a daily basis. The earth has become a toxic dump and poisonous substances have permeated our water, air and food. Somehow, our bodies must find a way of dealing with these toxin-loaded necessities of life. The immune system becomes overloaded when it is assaulted by too many toxins, and dysfunction is the result. Alternative medicine researchers and physicians believe that heavy metal poisoning is a major factor in autoimmune disorders, especially multiple sclerosis.

Different heavy metals have different routes of entry into the human system, yet all are devastating to the immune system. Cadmium, mercury, lead, arsenic, nickel and aluminum are the main heavy metals that are commonly found in human tissues at unacceptable levels. Heavy metals do most of their damage to our immune systems, rendering them defenseless against pathogens. How do heavy metals find their way into our bodies? We are exposed to lead through leaded gasoline, canned food with leaded seams, milk and meats from animals fed contaminated food, and leaded paint, for example.

Mercury, a potent neurotoxin, is found mainly in fish, especially canned tuna fish, and mercury amalgam dental fillings (silver fillings in your teeth). Having your mercury amalgam fillings removed is especially important to those with autoimmune diseases. However, North American dental associations refuse to admit that there is a connection between certain autoimmune diseases such as multiple sclerosis and mercury poisoning. Anecdotal cases of remission after removal of amalgams are reason enough to have these fillings replaced.

Cadmium exposure through cigarette smoke is the main reason for toxicity of this metal. Fertilizers, fungicides, rubber and paint are also common sources. Smoking cigarettes not only increases your chance of contracting lung cancer; it also exposes you to more than 6,000 chemicals, all of which need to be detoxified by the body.

Arsenic, one of the most toxic heavy metals, is found in herbicides and insecticides, paint and cigarette smoke. Arsenic is also found in the tips of the needles of coniferous trees, and arsenic poisoning has been seen in forestry workers and tree planters as well.

Aluminum is probably one of the most common heavy metals that we are exposed to. Aluminum sulphate is used by water-purification plants to remove impurities, such as clay particles, from our water. Studies conducted in France found there is a direct connection between Alzheimer's disease and traces of aluminum in tap water. This neurotoxin is also found in antiperspirants, baking powder, stomach antacids, aluminum household pots, pans and foil, and it is also prevalent in many laxatives.

Nickel is another heavy metal that in minute quantities is required in the body, but when exposure is too high, nickel toxicity results. Nickel exposure through dental appliances, including braces, can cause allergic reactions and immune dysfunction. Children who have just had their braces attached have a higher incidence of appendicitis than children without braces. The link has yet to be explained.

Chelation Removes Heavy Metals

Protection from exposure to heavy metals is important, but like most of us you have probably been exposed to these common heavy metal sources over your lifetime without even knowing it. High-dose antioxidants act as oral chelators, especially vitamin C and reduced L-glutathione, which help the body deal with free radicals and increase detoxification via the liver and kidneys. Chelate means to latch on to. In the case of heavy metals, the chelator attaches to the metal, carries it into the blood, then on to the kidneys to be excreted via the urine.

Intravenous chelation uses agents such as EDTA, DMPS, penicillamine or vitamin C directly into a vein. IV chelation is very effective at attaching to the heavy metals mentioned above, along with minerals that have been deposited in the blood and on the walls of arteries and veins. Although chelation will also remove other minerals along with the bad guys, your chelating physician will return these to your bloodstream to ensure adequate levels. Chelation is especially important in helping to detoxify those with autoimmune disorders so that the total toxic load can be reduced, allowing the immune system to function appropriately without an extra burden. Most individuals feel better within several IV chelation treatments. For those who are having their mercury amalgam dental fillings removed, chelation therapy can accelerate the mercury detoxification process.

DIABETES

Diabetes is a health epidemic. According to the Canadian Diabetes Association, over 100 million people are afflicted with diabetes worldwide. Over six million people are afflicted in the United States and in Canada. According to the U.S. Department of Health and Human Services, diabetes is the seventh leading cause of death.

When a person is diagnosed diabetic, it means that they either secrete little or no insulin, a reduced amount of insulin and/or their body does not respond appropriately to insulin, that is, it cannot transfer glucose from the bloodstream into cells and maintain blood glucose balance. Normally after we eat food, our blood sugar levels rise as we absorb glucose into the bloodstream. This causes the pancreas to produce insulin in order to return blood sugar levels to a normal range.

Insulin is a hormone secreted by the beta cells of the islets of Langerhans of the pancreas. It is essential for the metabolism of glucose by cells and is used in the treatment and control of diabetes mellitus.

Blood sugar is the glucose in the blood. It is measured in milligrams per 100 milliliters of blood.

Diabetes is categorized into two main types: Type I diabetes, commonly known as insulin-dependent diabetes mellitus (IDDM), affecting approximately 10 percent of all diabetics. Type II diabetes, or non-insulin dependent diabetes mellitus (NIDDM), affects 90 percent of diagnosed diabetics. Diabetes is still associated with a high rate of death resulting from its complications even though insulin-regulating treatments have advanced.

Diabetes is a serious disease that carries with it dangerous complications:

- eye diseases such as cataracts and retinopathy, which lead to blindness;
- kidney damage;
- neuropathy (nerve damage) results in numbness and pain in the hands and feet;
- hormonal imbalances due to the excessive production of cortisol, adrenaline, and sometimes insulin. All of these hormones reduce production of beneficial hormones such as DHEA;
- skin lesions and ulcers (especially in the legs where circulation becomes compromised). As a result, many diabetics must have leg amputations because leg ulcers progress and infection and gangrene take root;
- diabetic hypoglycemia is a particular risk for Type I diabetics taking insulin and for Type II diabetics taking insulin or sulfonylureas (drugs which increase insulin production); and
- increased risk of peripheral vascular disease, heart disease and cerebrovascular disease.

Type I Diabetes (Juvenile Onset Diabetes)

Unlike other autoimmune disorders, Type I diabetes affects both men and women equally. The disease is usually diagnosed around puberty and is often referred to as insulin-dependent juvenile diabetes. Type I diabetics need insulin because their pancreas produces little or no insulin due to the destruction of pancreatic insulin-secreting cells (B-cells) by the immune system. Over 80 percent of Type I diabetics have antibodies to their own pancreatic cells. Blood sugar levels must be monitored carefully and insulin is supplemented either through injection or intravenously.

The inability of the pancreas to produce insulin causes glucose to build up in the bloodstream and be excreted via the urinary system. Because glucose is not transferred to the cells, the body "starves" to death. Symptoms include excessive thirst, abnormal hunger, increased urination and weight loss.

Recent clinical studies indicate that infants who are breast-fed appear not to develop Type I diabetes as severely as those fed a cow's milk formula. Researchers believe that cow's milk protein, albumin, triggers an autoimmune reaction against the pancreas and causes the beginnings of its destruction. In addition to the cow's milk hypothesis of pancreatic autoimmune destruction, researchers also believe that viruses play a causative role in the development of Type I diabetes. Whooping cough virus, hepatitis, rubella, coxsackie, Epstein-Barr, cytomegalovirus and herpes virus are thought to induce autoimmune reactions in the body.

In addition to the complications listed above, Type I diabetics are particularly prone to ketoacidosis as a result of excess glucose buildup in the bloodstream. Without adequate insulin intake, a Type I diabetic will develop this dangerous condition whereby the body must break down fats for energy, causing excessive amounts of ketones to be produced. These ketones are deadly to the body as they allow acidosis to set in, which causes digestive and nervous system disorders. Insulin must be given under strict medical supervision to overcome this dangerous situation.

Type I diabetics are usually thin and have difficulty maintaining their weight. Moreover, the symptoms of Type I diabetes tend to occur very quickly and severely. In contrast, the symptoms of Type II diabetes occur gradually over a period of time. This is why many people who experience the symptoms of Type II diabetes may not realize they are developing the disease.

Type II Diabetes (Adult Onset Diabetes)

The majority of Type II diabetics tend to be over the age of 40 and overweight. More than 80 percent are obese; hence the reason that Type II diabetics can be further divided into obese and non-obese categories. Obesity is the number-one risk factor for developing this type of diabetes, and thinness is a prominent protector against the disease.

In Type II diabetes, although the pancreas may produce low or normal amounts of insulin, the peripheral organs and tissues have become resistant to insulin's effects. Food intolerances as well as viral infections can also cause lower insulin levels in Type II diabetes, increasing inflammation and encouraging autoimmune reactions to pancreatic cells. Fluctuating insulin levels are also caused by stress. Cortisol release by the adrenal glands increases the activity of antibodies and immune factors that increase inflammatory responses. Stress reduction, elimination of offending foods and fast treatment of viral diseases will help control insulin levels.

The symptoms of Type II diabetes appear gradually over years. So insidious are these symptoms that most people do not notice them creeping up. Symptoms include increased urination, abnormal thirst and excessive hunger, blurred vision, drowsiness, nausea and decreased exercise tolerance. As mentioned above, Type I diabetics develop a serious side effect of the disease called ketoacidosis. In contrast, Type II diabetics rarely develop this metabolic abnormality which is the reason why Type I diabetics are commonly thin and Type II diabetics are predominantly overweight. Due to risk factors such as smoking, obesity, hypertension and heredity, Type II diabetes is a serious health risk today.

Diagnosing Diabetes

For a positive diagnosis of diabetes, the National Diabetes Data Group of the National Institutes of Health advises the following test values:

- upon an overnight fast, blood glucose (blood sugar) levels greater than or equal to 140 milligrams per deciliter (mg/dl) on at least two separate measurements; and

- upon ingestion of 75 grams of glucose, blood glucose levels greater than or equal to 200 milligrams per deciliter (mg/dl) at two hours post-ingestion and at least one other sample during the two-hour test.

Diabetic Complications

Complications that arise for both Type I and Type II diabetes are a result of long-term elevations of either glucose or insulin. If blood glucose levels and blood insulin levels are allowed to vary outside of normal levels for extended periods of time, inflammation results and complications including nerve damage, blindness, kidney disease, heart and circulatory problems occur.

Sterols and Sterolins in Diabetes Treatment

In over 85 percent of cases of Type I diabetes, an autoimmune process is the cause of pancreatic cell destruction and an inability of the pancreas to produce insulin. Sterols and sterolins inhibit the secretion of interleukin-6, a powerful inflammatory factor, and decrease the action of B-cells to produce antibodies against its own tissues. In the remaining cases of Type I and Type II diabetes, sterols and sterolins work to control inflammation, thus reducing nerve damage, kidney failure and infections.

If you are on insulin therapy, careful monitoring of your blood glucose and blood insulin levels should be adopted. Insulin-dependent diabetics (Type I) will find that they require less insulin as a result of sterols and sterolins.

Sterinol does another important job—normalizing elevated cortisol levels and increasing subnormal DHEA levels. Because high cortisol and low DHEA accompany many cases of elevated insulin in patients with Type I and Type II diabetes, normalizing the DHEA-to-cortisol ratio will reduce high insulin levels in the blood and thereby signal the liver to reduce the production of acute phase inflammatory proteins. Sterols and sterolins are natural precursors to DHEA.

Dietary Changes

Dietary changes are an absolute priority for diabetics. The most important dietary changes to make for patients with carbohydrate metabolism disorders are:

- eat smaller and more frequent meals consisting of lower glycemic index foods (see below);
- eat more dietary fiber and nutrient-dense foods; and
- eat the appropriate foods for your blood type.

The glycemic index is a measure of a food's ability to increase blood glucose and insulin levels. Both types of diabetes respond well when frequent, small meals consisting of foods that only slowly increase blood glucose and insulin levels are consumed. For example, white bread is used as the standard for measurement of glycemic index and is assigned a glycemic index of 100. Ideally, better food choices involve eating lower glycemic foods such as legumes, vegetables and lean sources of protein. The glycemic index should not be the sole method of choosing foods because some very unhealthy foods (such as ice cream) have low glycemic indexes. Generally, however, healthy food choices and understanding the glycemic index will reduce sharp elevations in blood glucose, insulin, adrenaline and cortisol, allowing the body a chance to heal.

In addition to glycemic index considerations, attention should be paid to the level of dietary fiber in the diet. The ideal type of dietary fiber to consume is water-soluble plant fibers since they prevent rapid rises in blood sugar and improve tissue sensitivity to insulin. Good examples of water-soluble fiber include beans, most vegetables, and fruits such as apples and pears.

An emphasis on low glycemic and high fiber foods, in combination with eating the correct foods compatible with blood type, is a powerful method of promoting systemic healing. With the recent publication of his book *Eat Right For Your Type*, Dr. Peter J. D'Adamo continues and scientifically validates the concepts first proposed by his father, James D'Adamo. The concepts of the blood type program are scientifically validated and have been employed by many physicians in recent years to help sick patients become well. There are four basic blood types: O, A, B and AB, each different from the other due to structure of the blood type identifiers on red blood cells (called blood type antigens). Blood type antigens are immune system antigens and, as a result, will provoke an immune reaction called agglutination (clumping) in response to incompatible blood antigens. Because blood type antigens will mount a response to incompatible blood type antigens, a doctor must know your blood type in order to do blood transfusions, the wrong blood type could kill you.

In addition to reacting to incompatible blood type antigens, these antigens will also react to specific proteins in foods called lectins. Lectins are used as glues in nature. For example, bacteria in your intestinal tract use lectins to attach themselves to your bowel wall, and your body uses lectins to catch bacteria and parasites. Lectins in food that are incompatible with your blood type antigen will target a body system or organ and begin to agglutinate blood cells in that area. Because of this scientifically documented phenomenon, eating the proper foods for your blood type will significantly reduce agglutination and the risk of initiating an inflammatory/immune reaction. With respect to diabetes, Dr. D'Adamo states that Type I diabetes is much more common in blood type A and type B. Furthermore, he states that Type II diabetes often results in blood type O's who have eaten dairy, wheat and corn products over the years, and in blood type A's who have habitually consumed too much meat and dairy foods.

Nutritional Supplements Beneficial in Diabetes

Gamma Linolenic Acid

Gamma linolenic acid (GLA) is a fatty acid metabolite formed by the body from the omega-6 fatty acid family (safflower oil, sunflower oil). GLA is important in the body because it leads to the formation of vital local hormones called prostaglandins (specifically, prostaglandin E1). In times of nutritional deficiency, stress, viral diseases, diabetes and hypoglycemia, the formation of GLA is compromised or its utilization is increased and a relative deficiency may result. Consequently, supplementing with preformed gamma linolenic acid is preferrable rather than ingesting omega-6-rich oils and hoping that the body will create GLA from it. Some of the signs of GLA deficiencies include skin disorders, immune deficiency and nerve conduction problems. In diabetics, peripheral (arms and legs) nerve function is commonly impaired, resulting in loss of sensation and pain.

Controlled clinical trials using evening primrose oil (a highly effective source of gamma linolenic acid) demonstrated significant improvement of diabetes-related peripheral nerve dysfunction. Abnormal blood glucose and insulin levels severely lowers the activity of the enzyme responsible for forming GLA from dietary linoleic acid (omega-6 essential fatty acids) and, as a result, diabetics should be supplementing their diet with the most reduced form of essential fatty acids from evening primrose oil.

Efamol evening primrose oil should be taken with meals at a dosage of one 1000-mg capsule three times a day.

Eicosapentaenoic acid (EPA) and Docosahexanoic acid (DHA)

Both eicosapentaenoic acid (EPA) and docosahexanoic acid (DHA) are metabolites of the omega-3 fatty acid families. Fish oil is important in the body because, similar to the ingestion of GLA, it leads to the formation of prostaglandins as well (prostaglandin E3 in this case). Ingestion of fatty cold-water fish improves many of the abnormalities seen in diabetes. More specifically, fish oil lowers blood pressure, increases the level of "good" cholesterol (HDL cholesterol), reduces the level of "bad" cholesterol (LDL cholesterol) and lowers the levels of a protein that makes blood thicker and stickier (fibrinogen). Clinical trials using fish oils have been controversial since most commercially available fish oil supplements are unstable at room temperature. As a result, ingestion of these rancid oils results in increased production of free radicals in the body and side effects such as kidney toxicity and increased risk of coronary heart disease. In addition, commercial fish oil preparations contain high levels of chemical residues such as PCBs, known to cause adverse effects in even low amounts. Foods may be the best choice over supplementation. Fatty fish ingestion may help diabetics, but poor-quality fish oil supplements may be harmful.

Fortunately, not all fish oil supplements are bad. Based on extensive scientific analysis for levels of rancidity and harmful chemicals and clinical trials for efficacy, one fish oil preparation has demonstrated no detectable levels of harmful chemicals or rancidity—Eskimo-3 fish oil manufactured by Cardinova of Sweden. In fact, of 14 major brands of commercial fish oils tested, the Cardinova brand demonstrated room temperature stability for over 220 days, whereas other commercial preparations went rancid after approximately 21 days. Therefore, for the diabetic who wants the cardiovascular protective effects of fish oil, we recommend only the fish oils sold under the brand name Eskimo 3. (See Appendix I.)

Take one fish oil capsule 3 times daily or consume one 250-g portion of fatty fish such as salmon, herring or mackerel.

Reduced L-Glutathione (GSH)

Glutathione, composed of the amino acids glycine, glutamine and cysteine, is the most abundant intracellular antioxidant in mammalian tissues (see chapter 3). Glutathione exists in two forms in cells—the oxidized form (GSSH) and the reduced form (GSH). If the cell is going to use glutathione as an antioxidant to regenerate its used (oxidized) vitamin C or used vitamin E, the glutathione it contains must be able to donate electrons to these other molecules. Only glutathione in its active state (reduced) can accomplish this. In fact, a healthy cell always contains more reduced glutathione than oxidized glutathione. A reversal of this ratio is characteristic of sick cells because cell function crucially depends upon the proper ratio of GSH to GSSH.

In diabetics, supplementation with reduced L-glutathione (not L-glutathione) from between 500 mg to 2000 mg daily, in divided doses between meals, is crucial in management of diabetes and its complications. At this dosage level, GSH will prevent depletion of intracellular glutathione stores and the consequent free radical damage to cell membranes and cellular structures. In other words, the cell continues to function normally even in the presence of stressors. For the diabetic, this means that in spite of imbalanced insulin levels, glucose levels and hormonal levels (DHEA, cortisol, adrenaline, etc.), cells making up delicate tissues such as the eyes, nerves, pancreas, liver and circulatory system can function well and begin to repair themselves. In addition, supplementation with GSH has demonstrated the ability to increase a diabetic's insulin sensitivity.

Vitamins

Because of the metabolic disturbances inherent with disorders of carbohydrate metabolism, a diabetic will run the risk of major deficiencies in both fat-soluble vitamins (especially vitamin E) and water-soluble vitamins (especially vitamin C, niacinamide, biotin, vitamin B_{12} and vitamin B_6). The following key vitamins will benefit the diabetic:

- Vitamin E in a dose of 800 IU to 1200 IU will improve insulin sensitivity, glucose tolerance and will provide significant antioxidant protection for cell membranes. In fact, doctors who supplement their patients with essential fatty acids recommend increased intake of vitamin E in order to protect these beneficial fatty acids from becoming destroyed once incorporated into cell membranes;

- Because insulin is required for the transportation of vitamin C into the cell, diabetics are frequently deficient in vitamin C even if their diet is high in this important water-soluble vitamin. In addition to preventing deficiency states, a diabetic should supplement with vitamin C to bowel tolerance (see page 33) in order to take advantage of clinically documented effects of vitamin C in diabetics such as the reduction of sorbitol levels in sensitive tissues (such as red blood cells and eyes) and the inhibition of protein glycosylation. The vitamin C preparation ingested should be buffered for pH (in other words, the supplement should be near neutral in pH) and should replace vital trace elements such as manganese, copper and zinc.

It is important that insulin-dependent diabetics are carefully monitored by their physician whenever they are introducing new health regimens. Moderate exercise, along with an excellent nutritional program and the addition of diabetic-specific nutrients, will help control insulin levels and promote healing. As mentioned above, sterols and sterolins have the ability to modulate the immune system and reduce the serious complications associated with diabetes.

FIBROMYALGIA: THE INVISIBLE ILLNESS

Fibromyalgia (FM) is a common rheumatic syndrome that affects close to 7 million North Americans. The term "fibromyalgia" comes from the Latin words for *fibro*, meaning supportive tissue, *myo*, muscle, and *algia*, for pain. This disorder accounts for 15 to 30 percent of all visits to rheumatologists in North America. Like rheumatoid arthritis, fibromyalgia is more common in women than men and affects those between the ages of 35 to 60.

Diagnosis is Difficult

Fibromyalgia is called the invisible illness because it is so difficult to diagnose. It is characterized by musculoskeletal pain, stiffness and chronic aching. The most prominent symptom in this multisyndrome disorder is widespread muscle pain.

The pain is thought to be caused by a tightening and thickening of the thin film of tissue that holds muscles together. When diagnosing fibromyalgia, the physician applies pressure to certain trigger points including the neck, rib cage, hips, knees and shoulder area. For a diagnosis of FM, 11 of 18 specific locations must be tender.

Other symptoms of FM include allergies, anxiety, mental confusion, fatigue, carpal tunnel syndrome, depression, dizziness, heart palpitations, dysmenorrhea (painful menstrual cycle), fingernail ridges, stiffness, inability to exercise, gastrointestinal disturbances, headaches, sensitivity to light, sound and smell, mood swings, sleep disturbances, tender skin, total body pain and joint swelling. FM sufferers describe a feeling of extreme muscle fatigue as if they had been shoveling snow or gardening for days with no break. The pain is so extreme, they report, it feels as though their muscles are being stretched and torn. Each person has symptoms unique to them, making FM difficult to diagnose. Many diagnostic tests—blood, urine, X ray, CAT scan, magnetic resonance imaging (MRI), and more—may be performed with no conclusive evidence that there is anything wrong with the person. FM sufferers are often referred to psychiatrists for their symptoms. Moreover, it is often difficult for family and friends to understand the disease. Life becomes unbearable for those living with this painful condition, especially when no one takes their pain seriously.

What Causes FM?

There is no single cause for fibromyalgia. It is believed that multiple stressors, a traumatic emotional event, and stress and depressive episodes are major factors in the development of FM. Nutritional deficiencies and heavy metal and chemical toxicity also contribute. There is thought to be a connection between chronic fatigue syndrome (CFS) and FM as those who acquire FM often have a history of relentless fatigue. Repressed emotions or a traumatic emotional or physical event and serious illness are also linked to the disorder. Physicians must peel away the causal layers of each symptom and treat each one individually in order to deal with the disorder.

Treatments for Fibromyalgia

As mentioned above, many of the symptoms of FM overlap with those of chronic fatigue syndrome. The only difference between the two disorders is fatigue in CFS and muscle pain in FM. The recommendations for treating chronic fatigue syndrome (chapter 11) also apply to FM: adopt the immune system cure diet; detoxify your body; and eliminate your intake of and exposure to allergens.

Focus on repairing disrupted sleep patterns. Gentle exercise during the day (see page 151) and the addition of valerian extract or melatonin at night before retiring will help induce a restful sleep. Laughter has a beneficial action as mentioned in chapter 6 and along with exercise, both activities increase brain serotonin levels known for reducing pain. Moreover, gentle exercise not only helps to produce a good sleep state, it also enhances the function of the immune system. Poor sleep quality and pain go hand in hand with fibromyalgia. When one improves so does the other.

Take melatonin beginning with .5 mg and increase your dose until you obtain deep sleep without a groggy feeling the next day. Each person's dose is different, but on average around 10 mg is effective. Valerian also induces a relaxed, sleepy state. It is available in tablet, tincture and tea form. Choose the form you wish and take as recommended on the label.

5-HTP and St. John's wort are effective at increasing brain serotonin levels. In clinical trials, 5-HTP was shown to reduce symptoms of anxiety, muscle pain, disturbed sleep patterns and early-morning stiffness, as a dose of 100 mg three times a day. St. John's wort has been found to be effective in the treatment of depression. A dose of 100 mg, three times a day, is effective at reducing certain symptoms of FM.

As mentioned in chapter 3, magnesium is a potent immune-enhancing nutrient. Deficiency of this mineral is linked to many modern-day illnesses, FM being one of them. Magnesium is low in most chronic illnesses and is found in high concentration in muscle cells as it is required for production of ATP, the energy substance. This nutrient should be supplemented in a dose of 100 mg, three times a day. Magnesium glycinate is our choice as it is very well absorbed. Studies have shown that the combination of 300 to 600 mg of magnesium daily, along with malic acid, reduces FM symptoms.

Add a daily dose of malic acid to your immune system cure treatment program, 1200 to 2000 mg, as it is a powerful detoxifier of aluminum (see page 82 for more info on aluminum) and has been shown to reduce the pain associated with FM. Along with coenzyme Q_{10} (300 mg per day) and L-carnitine (500 mg per day) both are important for energy production.

Sterinol and Fibromyalgia

Chronic viral and bacterial infections are common in FM sufferers due to their compromised immune systems. Sterols and sterolins are highly effective at modulating the immune system and reducing inflammatory responses and autoantibody reactions. (See sterols and sterolins and rheumatoid arthritis in this chapter to understand the effectiveness of the plant fats in treating rheumatic conditions.) Be sure to make Sterinol the basis for your

FM recovery program—1 capsule three times a day on an empty stomach. Combined with the above additional nutrients, a good diet, detoxification methods, super-immune nutrients and phytonutrients, fibromyalgia will only be a bad memory.

Stefan Kuprowski, ND and director of the Ecomed Wellness Clinic, treats many FM patients and believes that FM is a curable condition. It requires a person to take responsibility for their own healing, he says; to seek the right professional help and therapies; and to see the illness not as a curse but as an opportunity for growth and self-transformation. No small task, but that is what is required to heal. Kuprowski maintains that since there are multiple causes to this illness, there are multiple cures. What works for one person may not work for another. Do not give up. The most important gift is the power of faith—faith in the healing process and faith in oneself to heal.

RHEUMATOID ARTHRITIS (RA)

Almost 50 million North Americans suffer from some form of arthritis. This group of diseases is so prevalent that mistakenly it is now considered a normal part of aging. Most individuals over the age of 55 have some signs of this group of diseases, whose common symptoms are pain, inflammation and varying degrees of joint stiffness and loss of movement of the joints.

Osteoarthritis, the most common arthritis, is recognized by damage to cartilage that covers and protects the ends of the bones in joints. Many of the recommendations for treating osteoarthritis are similar to those recommended for treating rheumatoid arthritis, with the exception of modulating the immune system. Osteoarthritis is not caused by a malfunctioning immune system, whereas RA is. Although we focus on RA when we make suggestions for the treatment and/or prevention of arthritis, we mean all forms of arthritis.

Rheumatoid arthritis is an autoimmune disease that affects more than 3 million people in Canada and the United States. People between the ages of 25-50 years old are most affected, and approximately 60 percent of those are women. In rheumatoid arthritis, the body's own defense system malfunctions and destroys healthy tissue. The synovial membranes, which cushion joint movements, are attacked, causing inflammation, and cartilage and bone destruction. If the disease's process is not arrested, joint deformity will result. RA most often strikes joints symmetrically, meaning it affects both sides of the body at the same time; for example, both wrists, both knees. Weight loss, fever, anemia, fatigue and general weakness often accompanies the painful joint inflammation. Blood tests are used to confirm the presence of rheumatoid factors.

Guidelines for Diagnosing Rheumatoid Arthritis

Four of seven criteria must be met for a diagnosis of rheumatoid arthritis.

- **morning stiffness**
  stiffness in and around the joints lasting one hour before improvement

- **arthritis of three or more joints**
  at least three joint areas, observed by a physician, simultaneously have soft tissue swelling or joint effusions, not just bony overgrowth, in the bones of the hands and feet, especially fingers and toes, wrists, ankles and elbows

- **arthritis of the hand joints**
  arthritis of wrist, hand bone and finger joints

- **symmetric arthritis**
  simultaneous involvement of the same joint areas on both sides of the body (i.e., both wrist joints, both knee joints, etc.)

- **rheumatoid nodules**
  nodules over bony prominences under the skin

- **serum rheumatoid factor**
  abnormal amounts of serum rheumatoid factor found by blood analysis

- **X ray changes**
  typical changes of rheumatoid arthritis on hand and wrist X rays, which must include erosions or bony decalcification

New Treatment for Rheumatoid Arthritis and Other Autoimmune Diseases

Research using Sterinol conducted at Tygerberg Hospital at the University of Stellenbosch and published in the *International Journal of Immuno-pharmacology* is providing an entirely new medical approach to the treatment of autoimmune diseases. Millions of people suffer from the destructive effects of RA and other autoimmune diseases. Sterinol offers new hope to those suffering from RA. Any treatment protocol for rheumatoid arthritis should be based upon the daily dosage of Sterinol plus some of the natural therapies discussed below.

Devil's Claw Root

At the beginning of the 20th century, European researchers discovered devil's claw root in Namibia, the former South West Africa. It was used as a folk remedy for the aged until it was proven to have therapeutic benefits in treating arthritic symptoms. Controlled clinical research in Europe compared the efficacy of a standard anti-arthritic drug, phenylbutazone, with that of devil's claw root. The results revealed devil's claw to be more effective in reducing pain and inflammation, and the root also produced no unpleasant side effects. One unexpected benefit was the relief of constipation.

Those who follow the devil's claw root regime find a reduction in pain and swelling within the first treatment course of three weeks; cholesterol and blood sugar levels also normalize. Interestingly, devil's claw root contains sterols and sterolins, which may be the reason for this root's anti-inflammatory properties. A remedial course of 3 tablets per day for three weeks is recommended.

Glucosamine Sulphate

Over a decade of research in Europe has shown that glucosamine sulphate is an effective treatment to repair damaged cartilage components around joints. Glucosamine normalizes cartilage metabolism while stopping its breakdown and thereby restoring joint function. The substance is an important constituent of bone and cartilage, skin, hair and nails.

Several studies have shown that glucosamine sulphate reduces pain and inflammation caused by arthritis-induced joint destruction. It also has the amazing ability to aid the rebuilding process of the cartilage matrix that makes up joint tissue. Researchers around the world have compared the effectiveness of glucosamine to the common pain reliever ibuprofen (Advil, Motrin and Nuprin, etc.). Double-blind, placebo-controlled studies verified that glucosamine was dramatically better at controlling both pain and inflammation compared to ibuprofen. Pain and inflammation were reduced even after the patient was no longer consuming glucosamine.

We recommend that you take Sterinol to stop the inflammatory process that is causing joint destruction, then add glucosamine sulphate to repair the damage that has already occurred. Although the research performed using glucosamine was performed on people with osteoarthritis, the resulting damage caused to the joints of rheumatoid arthritis is similar. RA is caused by an autoimmune disorder, whereas the mechanisms involved in osteoarthritis are quite different. Sterinol is effective at halting the joint-damaging process caused by autoantibodies, while glucosamine can repair damage already done to affected joints. Glucosamine sulphate at a dose of 500 mg, three times per day, is recommended. Cartilage repair usually begins within two months. Spectacular results have been experienced by those individuals with RA who have adopted the Sterinol, glucosamine sulphate regimen.

Chondroitin Sulphate

Chondroitin sulphate is a kind of natural body lubricant that provides cartilage with its elasticity and provides protection for bones in contact with one another, like a shock absorber. By halting the breakdown of old cartilage and stimulating the production of new cartilage, chondroitin sulphate is an effective treatment for the protection of joints. Again, as with glucosamine sulphate, many studies have confirmed the action of chondroitin. Long-term, placebo-controlled, double-blind studies performed in Europe found that chondroitin sulphate reduced pain and that damage to cartilage from arthritis was repaired to a significant degree within as little as three months. Again, even after the study subjects stopped taking the chondroitin, they experienced lasting effects into the post study evaluation period. Dr. Jason Theodosakis, author of *The Arthritis Cure*, recommends that chondroitin sulphate and glucosamine sulphate work synergistically to improve joint pain and inflammation. Chondroitin sulphate should be taken at a dosage of 400 mg, three times per day, in combination with glucosamine sulphate and Sterinol.

Fish and Flax: Healing Oils

Essential fatty acids (EFAs) from fish and flax oil are potent immune enhancers as well as powerful anti-inflammatory agents. EFAs form the lipid layer (allows the passage of substances into and out of the cell) of all cells in the body and control the development of the brain, eyes and nervous system. They also regulate prostaglandins that function to promote smooth muscle contractions and influence hormones. Omega-3 essential fatty acids are found in cold-water fish (herring, mackerel, salmon and tuna), flaxseed and walnut oil. Omega-6 essential fatty acids are found in canola, sunflower and safflower oils. Our diets are predominantly high in omega-6 oils from highly processed foods such as margarines and supermarket vegetable oils. Eliminate processed foods from your diet and add fresh, unrefined foods rich in essential fatty acids. Individuals who suffer from autoimmune diseases will notice how effective this simple diet change can be to the reduction of inflammatory symptoms.

Eicosapentaenoic acid (EPA) and docosahexaenoic acid (DHA) are made in the body from the omega-3 fatty acid alpha linolenic acid. EPA and DHA are found in high amounts in cold-water fish. These derivatives of the omega-3 fatty acids have powerful anti-inflammatory properties. Eat at least 3 to 5 servings of salmon, herring, mackerel and tuna each week. If you are unable to eat fish or dislike the taste, take one to three 500-mg capsules three times a day of either Efamol Marine or Tyler Eskimo 3 (see Appendix I).

Gamma Linolenic Acid (GLA)

Omega-6 fatty acids can be converted in the body to gamma linoleic acid (GLA) with the cofactors zinc and vitamin B_6. GLA has been found to inhibit the production of the inflammation-causing prostaglandins and leukotrienes that are overactive in autoimmune disorders. In one study, patients taking GLA from evening primrose oil were able to decrease their dosage of NSAID medication significantly and reported improved health compared to those in the placebo group. GLA has also been used in very high doses to eliminate the symptoms of multiple sclerosis.

Several randomized placebo-controlled, double-blind trials involving RA patients found that there was a significant reduction in both tender and swollen joints, and the need for pain medication was reduced along with inflammation upon supplementation with GLA. By down-regulating overzealous inflammatory processes, GLA is an effective treatment for autoimmune disease.

Take 3 tablespoons of flaxseed oil per day with 30 mg of zinc citrate and 50 mg of pyridoxal-5-phosphate with 100 mg of magnesium glycinate. It has been shown that many individuals, especially women, lack the enzyme to convert vitamin B_6 to its active form, pyridoxal-5-phosphate. As a result, we recommend pyridoxal-5-phosphate over vitamin B_6.

Dehydroepiandrosterone (DHEA): the Wonder Hormone

Dehydroepiandrosterone (DHEA) is reduced in people under stress and particularly in autoimmune disorders (see chapter 3). Studies show that DHEA reduces the number of antibodies attacking the "self" and therefore helps to control autoimmune disorders. Systemic lupus erythematosus research involving the effects of DHEA found that an unusually high dose of DHEA, 200 mg per day, reduced symptoms significantly. However, 200 mg per day should not be consumed without a physician's guidance. We recommend taking sterols and sterolins, as they naturally increase DHEA levels, helping to reduce inflammation and excess antibody production.

GENTLE EXERCISE FOR WEIGHT CONTROL

Our knees and hips bear up to ten times our body weight. Simply managing your weight and losing as little as 10 pounds can help to reduce the pressure your weight-bearing joints must carry. Begin with gentle exercise, nothing too strenuous. Here are some tips to keep your muscles and joints healthy:

- Walk every day, even if only to the end of your driveway and back. Take it easy, don't do too much. Walk 10 feet if that is all you can do.

- Join a beginner water-fitness class. These exercises are classed as "no impact" because the water provides you with a cushion. After your water-fitness class, sit in the sauna; you will benefit from some detoxification through your skin, and your joints will enjoy the warmth.

- Control your weight by eating plenty of fruits and vegetables, omitting the foods that are associated with increasing inflammation.

Nightshade family foods cause inflammation, and so do those that you are allergic to (see below). Inflammatory foods include milk, citrus and eggs.

- Eliminate all sugar from your diet.

- Do some weight-bearing exercises. Use light weights—half or one pound weights will do. We recommend Velcro weights you wear strapped around your legs or arms; they are very lightweight. An effective way to begin is to sit in a chair and lift your legs up and down, then lift your arms up and down—whatever works to get a little movement into your day.

- Rest and do not become fatigued.

- Find some activity you love to do, and do it as often as possible— gardening, walking, dancing, and so on.

ELIMINATE ALLERGIES

Allergies may be related to autoimmune diseases (see chapter 10). Elimination diets or blood tests can determine food hypersensitivities. Although never proven by formal research, approximately 10 percent of people who suffer from joint inflammation find their symptoms reduced when they eliminate foods from the nightshade family, including peppers, tomatoes, potatoes, eggplant, paprika and tobacco (cigarette smoking is out). Eliminating sugar, white flour, caffeine, citrus fruits and alcohol, and reducing red meat and dairy products also help many reduce the devastating effects of autoimmune diseases. Anti-inflammatory diets must limit red meat in order to decrease the levels of arachidonic acid, a powerful inflammatory agent.

Autoimmune states may be caused by delayed food sensitivities that cause leaky gut syndrome (or intestinal permeability problems), whereby undigested food particles are able to enter the bloodstream. Once in the blood, these particles are deposited into other body tissues where the immune system tries to eliminate them and inflammation results. A healthy intestinal lining is impermeable to antigens and toxins, but if the lining of the gut is compromised, the immune defenses must work overtime to keep invaders out. A leaky gut continually allows invaders to travel where they should not be, which will initiate an autoimmune response.

An article published in the *Canadian Journal of Physiology and Pharmacology* reported that celiac disease is a food allergy–induced autoimmune disorder, and it may well be that insulin-dependent diabetes mellitus is also related to food allergies. Research is under way to confirm the relationship between allergies and autoimmunity. If you are afflicted with an autoimmune disorder, allergy testing or eliminating suspect foods may help you get your symptoms under control.

MILK MAY NOT DO THE BODY GOOD

In an article published in *Healthy Living Guide*, world-renowned author (*The Atkins Diet Revolution*) and medical doctor, Dr. Robert Atkins wrote that according to some scientists, an infection is the primary cause of rheumatoid arthritis and that the infectious agent exists in milk. Researchers have also correlated higher levels of circulating anti-milk antibodies in those afflicted with RA. In the same article, Atkins suggests that the most effective dietary prescription to combat multiple sclerosis, developed by Dr. Hans Nieper, strictly forbids milk. Lab tests aren't conclusive yet, but some investigators believe that milk contains unknown toxic substances or that certain milk fats may somehow alter the nervous system.

CASE HISTORIES

NORMAN NEL

At age 32, I contracted rheumatoid arthritis. I had been through a very stressful period brought on by the financial risks of starting up a new business. As a married man with two young children at the time, I thought this condition would be disastrous to my short career. My doctor referred me to Dr. Anderson, a rheumatologist who confirmed my condition. I sought a second opinion and flew to Cape Town to see Professor Myers at Grootte Schuur Hospital who had no doubts about my condition and endorsed the previous diagnosis.

I was then put on medication (the trade name escapes me) but it was a cortisone-based pill for which I had an open prescription for repeat orders. The dosage was 1 tablet three times per day, and I continued to use this product for about two years. During that period, I developed lumps on my elbows the size of golf balls, and most of my finger joints were swollen, inflamed and painful to use. My wrists, knees and ankles were so badly affected that I could hardly walk. My weight dropped from 80 kilograms (172 pounds) to 65 kilograms (143 pounds). The doctors assured me that they would keep me out of a wheelchair as long as possible. They also cautioned me not to resort to iridologists (eye gazers), saliva analysts or "quacks," because if I did, they would not be prepared to treat me.

By chance, I heard through a friend about Mr. R. W. Liebenberg's natural product containing sterols and sterolins. I was told that the active ingredient was extracted from plants. I listened but I was reluctant to use anything other than what my doctors had prescribed. My long-time friend was clearly upset by the deterioration he was witnessing in my condition. He was persistent and I was at a low. My condition was wearing me down and I felt I had nothing to lose. I phoned Mr. Liebenberg and explained my condition to him. He invited me to his home office on an agricultural holding on the western side of the highway in Midrand, South Africa, where he gave me a free supply of capsules.

I swallowed those capsules faithfully, six to eight times per day. After about four months the pain eased. At first I was not sure because I continued to use the cortisone. I decided to gradually phase out the cortisone to make sure. To my absolute delight, the pain, swelling and inflammation had started to clear up. I continued to use the capsules for about three years (all supplied to me free of charge; Mr. Liebenberg appeared to have no profit motive whatsoever). My weight and health returned to normal.

I have just enjoyed my sixty-third birthday (October 22, 1998) and have used no medication whatsoever for the past twenty-five years. Looking at the only remaining distortion to my body, a slightly twisted front joint on my middle left-hand finger, to remind me that I once suffered from rheumatoid arthritis, I realized that it was time to give my heartfelt thanks to Mr. Liebenburg for the complete recovery that I have enjoyed. I can only hope this product is available to others.

I was told by my doctors that because medical science was not sure of the cause of rheumatoid arthritis, there was no cure. This statement is no longer true. There is a cure. It is sterols and sterolins.

Yours faithfully,

Norman Nel

DONNA BROOK

Dear Dr. Johan Lamprecht,

I am not sure if you remember, but I asked your advice for treating my son with systemic juvenile rheumatoid arthritis (JRA) with Moducare, Sterinol a couple of months ago. Well, here is a quick update on his condition. I have had him on half a capsule, three times per day since then. He was also on prednisone, 2 mg per kilogram per day, and Disprin. We weaned him off the prednisone after one month and have just stopped the Disprin as well, and he seems to be in complete remission. Dr. Power of the Red Cross says it is the most easily controlled case of JRA he has ever seen. Whether this is due to him starting the Moducare, who knows, but I am certainly not stopping it. Thought you might be interested to know the outcome of this treatment. Thank you for your help,

Donna Brook

LAURIE MARSHAM

Dear Lorna,

In October of 1997 I was diagnosed with lupus. My doctor wanted me to start taking steroids and anti-inflammatories. I did not want to go that route of treatment. With the help of friends, I was put in touch with a medical doctor who also practices natural medicine. I was having joint pain in my hands. They seemed to ache all the time, also pain in my hips that kept me awake at night. When I went to see him, I also found out that I had a problem with yeast, candida, wheat and gluten intolerance. I was put on large doses of acidophilus, and some other natural remedies. It seemed to help but I still had pain in my joints with considerable swelling. I started to take Moducare at the end of July and within 5 to 6 weeks my joints were aching less and less. I can now work in my garden without paying for it the next day. I hope next summer to be able to start playing golf again. Moducare (sterisol) is a wonderful product. I just wish more doctors would start taking notice of products like it so that more people can benefit the way that I have.

Laurie Marsham

ALLERGIES AND THE IMMUNE SYSTEM

Remember to cure the patient as well as the disease.

—Dr. Alvan Baruch

Twenty percent of the North American population is affected by an allergy to some normally inoffensive substance. Within this group most suffer from hay fever, rhinitis and asthma. Asthma, alone, accounts for a large majority of pediatric visits to hospital emergency rooms and 2 percent of total medical costs.

An allergy is the body's adverse reaction to a substance that to most people does not cause harm. These allergens include pollens, dust, dust mites, animal dander or other ordinarily benign chemicals and materials. Foods can also be a source of allergy in adults and children. Still other people are affected by allergic responses to insect stings or pharmaceutical substances. Allergic reactions include headaches, fatigue, sneezing, runny eyes, intestinal disturbances, skin rashes and more. They can contribute to rheumatoid arthritis, kidney disorders, pain, weight loss or gain, multiple sclerosis, diabetes, migraines and chronic bronchitis, among other disorders. In certain cases the immune system mounts such a serious assault on the offending substance that death is the result. Why would the immune system develop a defense that is potentially threatening to the very organism it is trying to protect?

WHAT CAUSES ALLERGIES?

Scientists have proposed an interesting hypothesis as to why the body responds to certain substances with an allergic reaction. It is believed that initially the immune system developed an allergic response to help the body deal with parasite infections. Survival of the fittest is the theory. People who could mount an effective response against parasite infections and survived had a greater chance of living a long life and bearing children. In areas of the world where parasite infection is common, this immune defense mechanism is very effective at ensuring survival, but in locations where parasites are not as prevalent, the body reacts more readily to not-so-dangerous invaders. Epidemiologists, scientists that study the incidence, distribution and control of disease in a population, argued that in developing countries allergic reactions are rare compared to developed countries, where they are common. This hypothesis was based on the understanding that everyday exposure to parasites is limited in developed countries and as a result the immune system is freed up to react to common substances.

The parasite theory has evolved even further with the realization that even in developed countries we are exposed to parasite infections more often than we realize due to increased air travel to foreign destinations, contaminated food and water and through sexual transmission. Parasite infection can cause severe damage to the intestinal lining, resulting in gut permeability problems and absorption of endotoxins, bacteria, yeast and undigested foods. Invasive damage caused by parasites does eventually lead to immune suppression and an increase in pro-inflammatory factors such as interleukin-6, which is responsible for the pain, inflammation and destruction seen in autoimmune disorders.

A parasite alert in the body causes the production of white blood cells that release factors which promote inflammation. This process is highly effective at calling other immune cells to arms, but it can also get out of hand in situations of chronic infection and damage the body's own tissues, resulting in pain and further inflammation as seen in many autoimmune conditions.

It is also believed that once the body has hit the limit of its toxic load (caused by overexposure to toxins), it malfunctions and is unable to distinguish clearly between substances that are not harmful and those that are. The immune system is seriously overworked dealing with the onslaught of environmental toxins it encounters every day. Antibiotics, hormone-altering drugs, mercury amalgam dental fillings, fluoride, chlorine and estrogen-laced plastics are only a few of the many chemicals we are exposed to. In *Non-toxic, Natural and Earthwise*, Debra Lynn Dadd states that the average North American consumes six pounds of chemicals annually. Our bodies are in a state of toxic overload. Furthermore, researchers who have studied the long-term effects of infant vaccinations believe that these inoculations may be linked to dysfunctions in the way the immune system views invaders or potential allergens. Although this has not been proven conclusively, it may be an important factor in allergy susceptibility.

IMMUNE RESPONSE INDUCES ALLERGY

Classic allergic response is marked by an increase in immunoglobulin E (IgE) antibodies that cause an immune system reaction promoting inflammation. When an IgE immunoglobulin encounters an invader, it triggers the release of chemicals from mast cells that can destroy or disable the offending agent. One of the chemicals released by mast cells as a result of IgE is histamine. Histamine is not only responsible for causing an allergic response, it is also a very effective parasite-killing agent—hence the allergy/parasite connection mentioned in earlier theories. IgE-mediated allergies are called atopic; for example, atopic eczema. These types of allergies usually run in families in one form or another.

Depending on the allergic response, different parts of the body are affected. We know that different allergens evoke symptoms by engaging the immune system at many sites in the body. An unruly immune response to pollens in the upper respiratory tract can result in sneezing and a runny nose (allergic rhinitis). The same pollen can cause an immune response in the lower respiratory system with symptoms such as wheezing or asthmatic reactions. It can also cause an immune reaction in the digestive system with symptoms of diarrhea, nausea, gas, pain or vomiting.

Anaphylactic Reaction

The most deadly reaction occurs when the allergen gets into the bloodstream and causes anaphylaxis, characterized by respiratory distress, fainting, itching, hives and often shock. The following substances are generally responsible for anaphylactic reactions:

- Venoms: wasps, bees, hornets
- Medications: hormones (insulin, parathormone), antibiotics (penicillin)
- Vaccinations: tetanus, diphtheria
- Foods: citrus fruits, mangoes, strawberries, nuts (Brazil, cashew), legumes (soybean, peanut), shellfish, chocolate

The earliest recorded anaphylactic reaction to an insect sting appears in the hieroglyphics of King Menes of Egypt 4,000 years ago. The term anaphylaxis, derived from the Greek meaning "anti-protection," was coined by two French biologists, Portier and Richet. They investigated whether prior exposure of dogs to sea anemone toxin would protect them from the severe reactions caused by the injection of anemone venom. To their surprise, the dogs died within 30 minutes of exposure to the venom after being sensitized to the toxin. This severe type of reaction often occurs on the second exposure to the substance, not the first. Insect stings, especially from bees, wasps and hornets, along with an allergy to penicillin, are the main causes of anaphylactic reactions. Many people die each year as a result of penicillin-induced anaphylaxis. Whatever the allergen, anaphylaxis is an emergency situation and treatment in the form of an injection of epinephrine (adrenaline) can combat the symptoms, opening airways and preventing death.

Types of Allergy-Immune Responses

There are two forms of allergic response: IgE-mediated and cell-mediated. A classic allergic reaction, such as one to shellfish, is very clearly IgE-mediated; reactions are of the fast-onset type and a simple blood test can confirm this. Some allergic reactions, however, are cell-mediated or IgG antibody–mediated and they do not follow the classic allergic symptoms, which makes them very difficult to diagnose. These include food intolerances or food sensitivities and they are often delayed, meaning that the symptoms may not appear rapidly, as in IgE-mediated allergic responses. IgG responses can cause an unusual group of symptoms not commonly seen in IgE-mediated allergies. These include gastrointestinal upsets, diarrhea and irritable bowel and brain fog type symptoms or hyperactivity, as seen in children. IgG reactions are also related to autoimmune disorders and may play a role in the cause of the immune system's unruly behavior.

Many people have IgG-mediated allergies and don't know it because their symptoms are vague. For example, a 40-year-old businessman with symptoms of fatigue and skin breakouts (mild acne) was not aware that he was severely allergic to wheat until he eliminated the offending foods. Once foods containing wheat were removed from his diet, he found that he no longer needed afternoon naps, his ability to solve problems improved and his skin cleared up. He felt like a new person and realized that he had been affected by this allergy since he was a child.

Children are affected similarly. How many children diagnosed with attention-deficit disorder and hyperactivity (ADHD) actually have IgG-mediated allergies that have not been discovered? Jason's story is a good example. A normally calm child at home, Jason started school, and within a few weeks his mother received a call from the kindergarten teacher saying that he was unruly and should be checked for ADHD. Symptoms of ADHD are an inability to focus and concentrate, hyperactivity, learning difficulties, behavioral problems, short attention span, sleep disturbances and emotional upsets. Jason's mother was surprised because at home he was peaceful. She attended several classes to observe her son's behavior and realized that something was causing Jason's symptoms. She noticed that Jason was the first to offer to clean the chalkboards; and he loved the classroom mascot, a guinea pig, which he could not wait to hold. The teacher also gave the children red licorice to reward appropriate behavior, and she was giving Jason this treat to encourage "good" behavior. Jason's mother was careful about nutrition and he had never consumed this type of candy until now.

After an appointment with the doctor to rule out ADHD and a consultation with the teacher, Jason was moved to the center of the room, as far away from the chalkboards as possible. The teacher stopped cleaning the boards during class time and the guinea pig was given away. With no more red licorice, Jason's behavior improved dramatically. This is an example of allergies that were not recognized, and through a concerted effort of the parent and teacher, the child avoided a misdiagnosis of ADHD and years of unpleasant symptoms.

It is possible that exposure to one allergen may not cause symptoms, but when combined with several offending substances the reaction becomes clearer. This is true with food allergies; wheat alone may only cause fatigue, but combined with dairy products, a compounded sensitivity will exacerbate symptoms. During hay fever season many people find they cannot eat certain foods because their symptoms worsen. Keeping a written diary of what you eat, where you have been and what you are exposed to will help you make the connections between situations and your allergies.

Eliminate Allergens

Although not often fatal, allergic conditions are extremely debilitating and can be very difficult to treat. Elimination of as many of the offending allergens is step one; adding the proper nutrients and nutrition will help support the body's healing process. Minimizing exposure to allergens will also help your immune system right itself and stop inflammation. This is especially true with food allergies, where the gastrointestinal tract is damaged and needs to be repaired. If the allergy-causing food is removed, inflammation will stop and the body will turn its attention to fixing the damage it has provoked.

Airborne allergens, particles that we breathe in, can cause allergic reactions. Dust mites, molds, pollens, animal dander, perfumes and other chemicals are some agents that cause allergy that must be eliminated, if possible, or their exposure must be reduced.

Offending foods, once discovered, should be eliminated for a period of six months. Then slowly, one by one, they may be replaced in the diet. Rotation diets, where the same foods are not eaten more than once a week, have also provided a reduction in allergic symptoms. Elimination diets are one method of determining allergy-causing foods. Rice, water and free-range chicken should be consumed for at least two weeks—nothing else. Then foods should be introduced as recommended for infants, one at a time—meaning one food each week. This is an extremely effective method of determining allergies to foods. Although it is difficult to follow, an elimination diet is well worth it in the end. Once you have determined your food allergies, a nutrition program should be designed to ensure you are getting adequate protein, vitamins and minerals.

As we have said, IgG- or cell-mediated allergies are not recognized by standard blood tests that test for IgE antibodies. As a result, your doctor might tell you that you do not have allergies. Russell Jaffe, Ph.D., has designed a test called the ELISA/ACT test which tests the presence of cell-mediated and IgE-mediated food allergies (see Appendix II). By doing this test, Lorna discovered that she had a delayed allergy to berries that was so severe it caused extreme hay fever symptoms during the berry season (June-July) in Vancouver. This test is well worth it if you have symptoms of varying degrees that are not related to any disorder. Fibromyalgia sufferers and persons with severe autoimmune disorders may want to rule out cell-mediated allergies.

Anatomy of an Allergic Response to Animal Dander

Allergy begins when the immune system discovers the presence of a harmless substance such as animal dander (bits of cast-off skin) and mistakes it for a dangerous invader. Urgently and swiftly, B-cells begin making IgE antibodies to destroy the foreigner. IgE causes the mast cells that line our nostrils to release histamine, serotonin, prostaglandins and leukotrienes that produce symptoms meant to eliminate the offender. A runny nose tries to eliminate the animal dander on a river of secretions; sneezing is another mechanism to rid the body and dislodge the invader; and then inflammation ensues to repair any area that has been exposed to the substance. All of the above are methods the body uses to evict an invader, and combined, cause an allergic reaction.

The first encounter of an allergen and the immune system often causes no allergic symptoms. It only sets the stage for a reaction when our defense system meets the allergen again. Macrophages take the allergen and break it down into fragments that are then presented to the body's T-cells. T-cells secrete interleukin-4 and then B-cells mature into plasma cells and secrete IgE antibodies. The antibodies then attach to mast cells and basophil cells. When two or more IgE molecules attach to the mast cell, a cascade of enzymes are released that induce inflammatory cytokines, which are responsible for the allergic reaction and the accompanying symptoms. Immune damage occurs when other defense cells migrate to the site of the allergic response. These recruited immune cells then release chemicals of their own that result in damage to tissue and the immune system.

Histamine is responsible for constricting bronchial airways, causing a difficulty in breathing and congestion in the respiratory tract. It also dilates blood vessels, which causes redness and inflammation. A lethal drop in blood pressure that can induce shock is a result of too much histamine being released into the bloodstream. Itching of the skin and pain are also caused by too much histamine. Leukotrienes, another immune system mediator, is also responsible for the constriction of airways and the swelling of tissue around the allergen entry site. Prostaglandins are also bronchial-constricting when released in excess. Combined, these mediators cause the host of allergic symptoms we are familiar with today.

Mechanisms of Hypersensitivity

- Hypersensitivity is the term used to describe the exaggerated or inappropriate immune responses that result in tissue damage.
- Allergy results from the activation of mast cells by IgE.
- An allergen is a small protein which, for unknown reasons, in some persons induces a persistent allergic response.
- The tendency to allergic reactions has a predominantly environmental basis.

Allergic Symptoms

It is easy to diagnose an allergy that presents itself quickly and clearly in the form of a runny nose and itchy eyes as a result of exposure to a particular agent such as cats or peanuts. It is much more difficult to discover an allergy that has vague symptoms or takes hours to display its effects. Symptoms can be severe or mild and can include:

- dark circles under the eyes
- red-rimmed or swollen watery eyes
- red burning ears
- runny nose
- constant nose rubbing (some allergic people have a crease just above the bulb of the nose from chronic rubbing, or one nostril will be stretched in the direction of the rub)
- inflamed tonsils and recurrent throat infections
- skin rashes, eczema
- diarrhea, gas, constipation, nausea, bloated stomach, heartburn and stomachaches
- excessive sweating
- headaches, dizziness

- extreme salivation
- joint and muscle pain
- fatigue
- poor memory or fogginess
- bed-wetting in children
- mood swings

ASTHMA

Asthma is the most common chronic childhood disease. It is characterized by increased respiratory distress of the bronchi with resulting airway narrowing, which is associated with inflammation. Wheezing and shortness of breath are the main symptoms. There are three main types of asthma. Extrinsic asthma is associated with high circulating IgE antibodies, is seasonal in nature, is not chronic, has childhood onset, a family history of allergy and positive skin allergy tests. Occupational asthma is different in that it is not always IgE-mediated and is generally caused by a hypersensitivity to chemical substances such as toluene and plastics. Intrinsic asthma affects adults and normal IgE levels are found to be present.

Fifty percent of all cases of asthma diagnosed today have an allergic component. Therefore, eliminating offending allergens is important in managing the disease. Pets, dust, foods, inhalants, and so on must be removed from the environment. Antihistamine drugs are not effective in the treatment of asthma and should not be consumed. Corticosteroid drugs are prescribed for those with moderate to severe symptoms for the ability of these medications to suppress the immune system.

Several studies have looked at airborne allergen exposure during infancy in relation to asthma and allergic rhinitis. It is very interesting that children raised in areas of low altitude have significantly higher rates of asthma. Moreover, children born during the high pollen months have a higher incidence of asthma and allergic rhinitis compared to those born during non-pollen production months. If you have a strong family history of asthma, choosing low pollen months for the birth of your child may be an important factor in protecting your child from future allergies.

In North America, where double-glazing windows, central heating and energy-efficient homes are the norm, an overabundance of dust mites and molds result, which exacerbates allergic diseases. Fresh air and a clean home will help minimize the risks of contracting allergies. One friend who had terrible mold sensitivities put a concerted effort into eliminating mold from his home but still had allergies. Eventually, he realized that the toilet-water holding tank was the source, and once this situation was remedied, his symptoms dissipated. His determination to get to the root of his allergies resulted in a complete remission of his symptoms.

A six-year-old boy we saw was taking high doses of corticosteroids to reduce his severe asthma symptoms. He was admitted to hospital no less than ten times each month with frightening episodes of reduced air intake. After three weeks on Sterinol along with bioflavonoids, his symptoms reduced so dramatically that he no longer was using the corticosteroids. At the same time, his parents had the carpets removed from their home, their furnace vents cleaned and all curtains taken out of the boy's bedroom. By reducing the allergen load and modulating their son's immune system with Sterinol, they were able to effect a positive change in the boy's symptoms.

Elimination of allergens, the inclusion of Sterinol, fish oils and bioflavonoids should be incorporated into a diet high in organic fruits, vegetables and legumes.

ALLERGIC RHINITIS

Allergic rhinitis may appear to be a minor allergy—unless you have suffered a nose that runs like a faucet. Annual medical costs for this seemingly trivial disorder amounts to over 500 million dollars in the United States. The condition affects up to 10 percent of children and 20 percent of teenagers and has an impact on the school performance of those afflicted. Symptoms include nasal congestion, sneezing, itching and discharge. The eyes can also be involved with conjunctivitis (mucus eyes), excessive watering, sensitivity to light, itching and a gritty feeling. Even an itchy palate on the roof of the mouth and throat are not uncommon. Middle-ear infections and fluid buildup are also symptoms. As mentioned above, a crease just above the bulb of the nose is a clear indicator of allergic rhinitis from chronic rubbing or wiping.

Common allergens such as seasonal pollens, pets, dust and chemicals create hyper-responsiveness by the upper respiratory system. Medical treatments center on over-the-counter antihistamines and allergen avoidance.

The latter is particularly difficult if the allergen is pollen or dust. Pyridoxal-5-phosphate has been found to heal mucosal linings. Intact nasal mucosa offer a physical barrier or first line of defense against invading allergens. Children should take 25 mg per day and adults 150 mg per day in conjunction with 15 mg of zinc citrate and 100 mg of magnesium glycinate. Ensure that environmental factors are cleaned up and eliminated. And adopt the immune-boosting diet recommended in chapter 5.

Preliminary results of a clinical trial in Cape Town, South Africa, determined that Sterinol is effective at alleviating the symptoms of allergic rhinitis. Three capsules daily was prescribed in this trial.

ALLERGIC ECZEMA

Eczema is the most aggravating of the allergic conditions. Extreme itching, red, dry patches with occasional vesicles (i.e., blisters) that are crusty are symptoms of the disorder. In infants, the cheeks, abdomen, arms and legs are affected. Older children have eczema patches in the creases of the elbows, knees and wrists. Dermatitis is the term often used interchangeably with the term eczema. Dermatitis is a catchall term for inflammation of the skin; eczema is an inflammatory condition of the skin characterized by redness, itching and oozing blisters, which become scaly, crusted or hardened.

Allergic eczema is a common disorder that affects between 5 and 10 percent of the population. Children under the age of five are most susceptible to it. Avoiding certain trigger foods such as cow's milk and eggs have brought about improvement of the condition in children, but not in adults.

Breast-feeding an infant provides a protective effect against allergies, especially eczema. Secretory IgA, found in breast milk, offers protection to an infant's gastrointestinal tract from allergens in the environment. Moreover, pregnant or nursing mothers should be aware that cow's milk proteins can cross the placenta to the fetus and have also been found unaltered in breast milk. If you have a family history of eczema, avoiding milk while pregnant or breast-feeding may offer protection to your infant.

HIVES AND RASHES

Urticaria is the term used for hives and rashes caused by allergy. Itchy, raised round patches can erupt over several areas of the body in response to an allergy. Angio-edema is a related disorder and is characterized by edema (an abnormal excess accumulation of fluid in connective tissue) within the layers of the skin (dermis). Both of these disorders are caused by IgE-mediated immune reactions. Food allergies to seafood, nuts, berries, eggs and chocolate are the most common cause of urticaria. Symptoms may also include tingling and swelling of the tongue and area around the mouth.

Insect stings and allergies to prescription drugs may also produce hives and rashes. This condition usually has a fast onset and is not long lasting. Avoidance of allergens is the most common-sense approach.

Care must be taken when introducing new foods to infants. If you have a family history of severe allergy to seafood or nuts, wait until your child is over the age of five before introducing the most offending foods. This may help reduce the likelihood of an allergic response.

Sterinol is especially beneficial in inhibiting IgE-mediated responses and therefore may help stop urticaria before it begins. Due to their anti-histamine action, bioflavonoids are also an excellent adjuvant to Sterinol.

CHEMICAL SENSITIVITIES AND ENVIRONMENTAL ILLNESS

Environmental illness, a disease unheard of 50 years ago, is a result of living in a chemical-laden world. It is hard to believe that someone could have a reaction to something like the smell of plastic or the odor of Teflon from a heated pan, but these are now common symptoms of this "modern" disease. Daily we are exposed to strange new chemicals found in our toiletries, soaps, shampoos, food packaging materials and so much more that it is no wonder our immune system has gone awry. Symptoms of chemical sensitivities are so broad they can include every system in the body—cardiovascular, immune, gastrointestinal, respiratory and endocrine.

Help Your Body Detoxify

Avoid chemicals that you are sensitive to. Diplomatically ask friends, family or business associates not to wear perfumes or aftershave lotions if it causes you problems. Avoidance is one approach, but detoxification of the body is especially important in overcoming your current symptoms and helping to handle those you are exposed to. The nutrients recommended in chapter 3 are important in detoxifying your body and boosting its immunity. Reduced L-glutathione is the most powerful eliminator of toxins, along with vitamin C. Other therapies that have proven effective in speeding detoxification include taking saunas, massage treatments, exercise, dry-brushing and oxygen therapies—hydrogen peroxide or ozone. Drink plenty of purified water while undergoing any of the above treatments.

Toxin-Eliminating Bath

Epsom salts and baking soda baths are also another quick way to eliminate toxins from your body and speed healing.

1 – 1-pound bag (500 g) Epsom salts (available at the pharmacy)

1 – 1-pound box (500 g) of bicarbonate of soda (baking soda)

Run a bath as hot as you can tolerate. Pour in the Epsom salts and baking soda. Dry-brush using a special brush you can buy at the health food store. Make sure you brush toward your heart, meaning from your hands to your shoulders, and from your feet to your hips and so on. Get in the bath and soak until the water feels cool. Towel dry. Rub sesame oil onto the soles of your feet, put socks on and then get into bed and rest until morning. Epsom salts are magnesium sulphate; as we learned in chapter 3, magnesium is necessary for many reactions in the body and we are often deficient in this mineral. It, along with baking soda, helps detoxify the body as well. Once you try this detoxification and stress-relieving treatment, you will wonder what you did without it.

MOTHER HAS ALLERGIES, WILL I?

Hereditary factors do set us up for a susceptibility to a disease, but that does not mean that we will be afflicted. A predisposition is a reason to ensure that you take adequate steps to protect your body from immune dysfunction and potential health problems. Allergies appear to run in families, and if both your mother and father have a severe allergy to wheat, you may have a higher than average risk of developing that particular allergy. Therefore, avoiding the potential allergen and protecting your immune system from undue stress and environmental toxins is a smart idea.

IMMUNOTHERAPY

Desensitization or immunotherapy using repeated injections of an offending allergen to desensitize the body can provide relief to some individuals. Increasing doses of the allergen are introduced until the immune response becomes decreased or the person becomes desensitized. This therapy is recommended for classical allergies or for those who are IgE mediated. Skin tests and a RAST (radioallergosorbent) test must show positive to confirm IgE-mediated production against the allergen. Those individuals with an allergy to insect stings that result in an anaphylactic reaction are good candidates for immunotherapy. It is unclear what mechanism is at work with desensitization therapy, but there are several theories: antibody production may be blocked; immune suppression may occur; immunotherapy may tip the balance of T_H1 to T_H2 cells in favor of the T_H1 cells, and a resulting decrease in IgE antibodies. Many allergy sufferers do quite well with this type of therapy; others do not respond at all. Interesting that immunotherapy provides the same effect as sterol and sterolin therapy in relation to T_H1 and T_H2 regulation. Sterols and sterolins also increase T_H1 activity and reduce IgE production, albeit naturally.

STEROLS, STEROLINS AND ALLERGIES

As mentioned above, the regulation of IgE production is under the control of T-cell cytokines. Researchers have found that when helper T-cells are prepared from allergic people and are then incubated (in a test tube) with the allergens to which they suffer an allergic response, these T_H2-type helper T-cells release interleukin-4, interleukin-5 and interleukin-6. Interleukin-4 induces the synthesis of IgE by the B-cells.

Gamma interferon is secreted by T_H1-type helper T-cells and is reduced during the allergic response, and can therefore not control the release of interleukin-4 by other helper T-cells. In a normal immune response, interferon is responsible for stopping the release of interleukin-4, thereby reducing the production of IgE antibodies. Sterols and sterolins stimulate the release of T_H1-type cytokines from helper T-cells and as a result control the allergic condition by decreasing the manufacture of IgE.

Sterols and sterolins also reduce the synthesis of interleukin-6, the inflammation factor. It is known that during the late phase of an asthma episode, interleukin-6 perpetuates the inflammatory response, which causes bronchial tissue damage. Hence, even during an asthma attack, sterols and sterolins can protect against inflammation, indirectly resulting in far fewer symptoms. A balance between T_H1 cells and T_H2 cells is of paramount importance in controlling allergic symptoms. Sterinol maintains that balance and improves immune health. Remember, allergy is an immune system mistake. By ensuring that the body's defense mechanisms are in balance, we can protect ourselves from the destructive effects of chronic allergic response.

Currently, a clinical trial is under way to confirm the anecdotal accounts of allergy remission. So far, individuals who have added sterols and sterolins to their treatment protocol have gained tremendous results in symptom reduction. Within thirty days, individuals suffering allergies from pollens, animal dander and foods have seen their allergic responses diminish. Although sterols and sterolins are not a cure for allergic conditions, they are a safe, inexpensive protective agent that eliminates the symptoms of allergy, with no side effects. It is believed that long-term elimination of symptoms will allow the body to heal itself, thereby teaching the immune system to respond appropriately to common substances such as food, dust and pollen.

Daily recommended dose of Sterinol is 1 capsule upon rising, 1 capsule in the afternoon and 1 before going to bed. Remember, sterols and sterolins should not be taken with animal fats, as their absorption is inhibited.

QUERCETIN: NATURE'S ANTIHISTAMINE

Quercetin is a powerful antiallergy nutrient capable of inhibiting inflammation. By halting the production and release of histamine and interleukin-6, allergic symptoms are reduced dramatically. Research has shown that quercetin, a potent flavonoid, has an antiviral action specifically against type-1 herpes virus, influenza and polio virus type-1. In test tube studies, quercetin has stopped the replication of viruses as well as their ability to infect cells. Quercetin has also been shown to inhibit the replication of the HI virus by 100 percent in vitro. Animal studies have further confirmed the action of quercetin to stop viral infections.

Quercetin is especially effective in reducing the symptoms of asthma and environmental allergies. It modulates allergic responses and hypersensitivity disorders. This very powerful nutritional ally inhibits the release of histamine and leukotrienes by strengthening the cell membranes of mast cells. The IgE allergic antibodies cause mast cell and basophil membranes to become leaky, which allows the allergy-promoting histamine and other cytokines to release into surrounding tissues and blood. Individuals who take quercetin daily have very regular shaped, solid cell membranes.

Basophils are a type of white blood cell involved in allergic responses. They are activated by the antibody IgE, and are called mast cells when they have left the bloodstream and entered the tissues. The basophil and mast cell membrane is the outer perimeter of the cell. If we were talking about plants, it would be the cell wall. But human cells do not have walls; they have membranes which keep the inside contents of the cell separate from the outside.

Quercetin is structurally related to the antiallergy drug disodium cromoglycate. These two compounds have the same mechanism of action in which they block histamine release through the inhibition of receptor-mediated calcium channels in mast cell membranes. Through this action, the influx of calcium is prevented and mast cells are unable to break down or degranulate.

One cause of asthma is the release of leukotrienes derived from arachidonic acid with the aid of the enzymes phospholipase A_2 and lipoxygenase. Quercetin inhibits both enzymes and is therefore effective at halting leukotriene synthesis. By reducing IgE-mediated responses and inhibiting the enzymes responsible for making leukotrienes, quercetin is an effective antiasthma nutrient.

An article entitled "Natural Antioxidants: Effects of N-Acetyl-L-Cysteine, Quercetin and Standardized Ginkgo Biloba Extract" states that quercetin is also a potent inhibitor of aldose reductase, an enzyme that promotes the synthesis and intracellular accumulation of sorbitol. Sorbitol accumulation is implicated in the cause of cataracts, retinopathies (noninflammatory disorders of the retina), neuropathies (degenerative states of the nervous system or nerves) and other disorders, due to its osmotic effects (the flow of fluid between semipermeable membranes until equilibrium is reached). Diabetic animals have been shown to be particularly prone to sorbitol accumulation. Human studies have shown quercetin to be effective in the treatment of complications secondary to diabetes (see chapter 9).

Vitamin C sparing (slowing the loss of vitamin C from the body) is enhanced when quercetin is supplemented at the same time, and it has also been found to be a potent antioxidant and free radical scavenger. It is anticarcinogenic and anti-inflammatory as well. We recommend 1,000 to 1,500 mg of quercetin per day to suppress allergic reactions and the inflammation of arthritis.

PROANTHOCYANIDINS

Like quercetin, proanthocyanidins are important bioflavonoids that have powerful antiallergy, antihistamine, antiviral and antioxidant properties. The tartness of a lemon, the bouquet of a fine red wine and the deep colors of fruits and vegetables are all a result of a combination of bioflavonoids. More than 4,000 bioflavonoids have been discovered to date. One of the most potent and well researched of the proanthocyanidins derives from the bark of the Maritime pine sold under the trademark Pycnogenol. Moreover, this special family of nutrients includes grape seed extract and bilberry (see chapter 4). To control histamine release and degranulation of mast cells, a dosage of six, 500-mg capsules of one of the above recommended proanthocyanidins is recommended.

Excellent results in the control of hay fever symptoms is obtained with the addition of Pycnogenol. Pycnogenol also improves joint flexibility and repairs connective tissue by reducing the production of the enzymes and "bad" prostaglandins that cause inflammation. It also inhibits histamine release responsible for further tissue damage.

Proanthocyanidins have antioxidant activity 50 times more powerful than vitamin E and 20 times more potent than vitamin C. These potent bioflavonoids patrol the body, protecting it from free radical damage, and they inhibit the oxidation of fats, the process by which fats turn rancid. LDL, low density lipoproteins, the "bad" cholesterol, are particularly vulnerable to damage caused by oxidation. Once oxidized, LDL cholesterol attaches to the arteries and plays a role in causing arteriosclerosis (hardening of the arteries). The Lancet published a study showing that with high intakes of bioflavonoids, elderly men experienced a lower risk of heart disease and heart attack.

FISH OILS CONTROL ASTHMA

An epidemiological study reported that eating fish as little as once a week reduced the risk of developing respiratory disease. A study of the association between diet and asthma in children showed that children who ate fresh, oily fish had a significant reduction in asthma symptoms. It was found that oily fish was the only food that had a profound impact on the effects of asthma. Another study found that dietary fish consumption was associated with better lung function when measured by forced expiratory volume (FEV), a test in which asthmatics breathe into a machine that measures how much breathing capacity they have. Fish oil also exerts positive effects on arachidonic acid metabolism. Arachidonic acid is responsible for making the "bad guy" prostaglandins that cause inflammation and aggravate the allergic symptoms of asthma, psoriasis, eczema and other related disorders. (Read more about essential fatty acids in chapter 5.)

A daily dose of 500 mg can be given to children under the age of 5; 1,000 mg for children between 5 and 12 years of age; and 1,500 to 2,000 mg for adults.

There is no need to suffer allergies when nature has provided us with such an array of effective remedies. Stress management techniques, allergen avoidance, good nutrition and immune-boosting and modulating nutrients will heal your allergies.

CASE HISTORY

Dear Lorna,

I want to thank you for Sterinol. It has made an incredible difference in a severe allergy I used to have to cats. My life has been changed forever. I have been plagued by animal allergies since childhood with symptoms so severe that I could not visit the homes of my friends who had animals.

I recently met a woman with whom I wanted to begin a relationship. When I visited her home I found that she had two beautiful cats that she loved very much. I knew I would have to stop seeing her because I could never have a relationship with someone who lived with cats.

It is unbearable to suffer my allergic symptoms: severe runny nose, burning eyes, wheezing and extreme fatigue were some of the reactions I endured. However, this time it was different. When my new friend learned of my allergy, she recommended I take Sterinol. I was skeptical, but willing to try anything. I had taken antihistamines in the past, but even the strongest variety did nothing to reduce the severity of my attacks, and they left me with a hungover feeling for days. After one week of Sterinol I could stay in the house for hours, and within two months the cats no longer bothered me on my visits to her home. I know that Sterinol is responsible [for the improvement] because when I miss one day, my symptoms return. This is a miracle as I have suffered these allergies since childhood.

I am very happy, because not only did I get rid of my allergies but I also found a woman I want to spend the rest of my life with. Thank you to Sterinol.

J. B.

INFECTIOUS DISEASES AND IMMUNITY

Healing is possible even when a cure is not.

—Bill Moyers

For centuries, infectious diseases have been the leading cause of sickness and death. Outbreaks of influenza, polio, malaria, bubonic plague, cholera and tuberculosis have resulted in suffering and loss of life. Entire communities have been annihilated or left devastated as the result of a bacteria or virus that effectively invaded the body. Antibiotic treatments and mass vaccinations, until recently, appeared to be effective at eradicating many infectious diseases, especially smallpox. Health authorities believed that the day would come when infectious diseases would not be a bane of our existence; that is, until the appearance of HIV, AIDS and antibiotic-resistant bacteria. Now we realize that antibiotics and vaccinations are not the panacea we hoped for. Research to find a vaccine to combat HIV has been difficult as this virus has devised a method to outsmart both scientists and the body's mechanism for eradicating it. Bacteria have also mutated to avoid the effects of antibiotic treatments.

We have bombarded our bodies with thousands of toxins, countless antibiotics, nutrient-poor foods and inordinate stress, all to the detriment of proper immune function. While we have been ignoring these factors that undermine our health, microorganisms have been evolving and mutating to circumvent our normal immune response. Normally, we would evolve to ensure our survival, not allowing invaders to get the best of us. Due to technological advances, we have polluted our environment and ourselves so quickly that our bodies cannot adapt fast enough to the many toxins it is exposed to, and we are falling behind in our evolutionary ability. If we want to survive through the millennium, we must get back to basics and put our immune system in balance.

The key to a successful battle against infectious organisms lies within the human immune system. Our immunological defenses meet countless and endless opponents every day, only succumbing to infection when measures and countermeasures fail to defeat invaders. Although bacteria, viruses and parasites have devised a variety of tricks to evade our defense system's armaments, our immune system is almost always victorious. The goal of these invaders is not to kill their host. This would not be in the best interests of their own survival, yet often this is exactly what happens when we do not properly take care of the body's protective mechanism.

Viruses range from mildly disruptive to life-threatening. Only people who are immune-suppressed need fear a cold virus, but most of us have a serious respect for microorganisms that develop hepatitis C, HIV, tuberculosis and malaria—all life-threatening diseases. How the immune system responds to these daunting challenges determines our very survival. You can deal with infection by any type of organisms by strategically combining all the warriors of the immune system in full force.

IMMUNE RESPONSE TO INVADERS

Antibodies produced by B-cells are especially effective at destroying bacteria that live outside human cells, whereas helper T-cells are important in defeating bacteria and parasites that manage to set up house inside our cells. These helper T-cells work by secreting substances that amplify and control the immune response. Yet another immune cell, the cytotoxic T-cell deals with viruses that have devised a way to use the operational machinery inside our cells. Each type of immune cell works interdependently in a highly sophisticated assault on pathogens.

How the Immune System Responds to Bacteria

Pneumonia is a common respiratory disease caused by infection from the streptococcus pneumoniae or pneumococcus bacterium. It enters the body via the lungs, and colonizes in the alveoli (small sacs) of the lungs. Upon multiplication this bacteria causes tissue damage and inflammation resulting in impaired breathing. If the bacteria are left to flourish untreated, serious complications can develop and the person may even die. We would think that because these bacteria live outside cells, the immune system would make quick work of destroying them, but like most pathogens, pneumococcus bacteria have devised a way to avoid detection by macrophages. By surrounding themselves with a coating, phagocytic cells (macrophages) cannot digest these bacteria. The immune system has solved this problem by using antibodies produced by B-cells that allow phagocytes a place to lock onto the bacteria and do their job. The binding of one antibody to a bacterium activates complement (see chapter 2) and a corresponding cascade of enzymatic reactions that break down and destroy the offender. Extracellular bacteria, such as the pneumococcus, are handled well by this simple antibody immune reaction when the body's defense system is operating optimally.

Parasitic and Viral Infections

The antibody reaction works well for pathogens that do not live inside cells. Once inside cells, parasites and viruses cannot be harmed by antibodies or the complement reaction as these mechanisms were designed for free-floating or extracellular invaders. As a result, the immune system had to develop another tactic to deal with this type of invasion. Before cellular infection occurs, prompt action by macrophages, natural killer cells and phagocytes deal with the invader, but once infection is completed, the T-cells provide the main line of defense.

There are two types of intracellular infections. In the first form of infection, microorganisms are found within membrane-bound organelles through which they entered the cell, including endosomes and lysosomes. Tuberculosis and leprosy are two bacteria that use this type of entry method. In the second form of infection, microorganisms access the cell through the fluid part of the cell. Viruses are the most common microorganisms to use this form of decoy to evade detection.

Organelles are the microscopic organs within cells. **Endosomes** are a structure within the cell. A **lysosome** is a membrane-bound organelle that contains enzymes that are capable of lysing or destroying cells.

When a parasite or virus gains access to the internal environment of the cell, the cell produces a substance called major histocompatibility complex (MHC) that provides fragments which are presented to the surface of the cell, notifying passing helper T-cells. Through this recognition process, the T_H1 helper cell releases the cytokine gamma-interferon, which prompts other cytokines, such as tumor necrosis factor and nitric oxide, leading to the destruction of the invading microorganism. When the immune system is not functioning appropriately, T_H2 helper cells may predominantly release the cytokines interleukin-4 and interleukin-10 and not gamma-interferon. These two interleukins inhibit the microorganism-killing ability of the immune response. It is clear that the cytokines the helper T-cells choose to release play an extremely important role in the ability of the immune system to stop infection and disease. This decision by the helper T-cells to release either T_H1 cytokines or T_H2 cytokines sets the stage for the body's ability to fight infection or succumb to it. This may be the reason that one person seems immune to certain pathogens whereas another succumbs.

Studies examining tuberculosis infection have found that people who are T_H1 dominant with the release of protective gamma-interferon have better outcomes than those who are T_H2-dominant and release interleukin-4 and interleukin-10.

Killing Intracellular Viruses

Viruses live in the fluid-filled interior of cells and interact with and use many components of the cell. For example, they use the protein-manufacturing aspects of the cell to make their own proteins necessary for reproduction. Although it makes it more difficult to seek and destroy viruses because of this adaptation, fortunately the immune system has circumvented these problems. Cytotoxic T-cells are enlisted to respond to virus-infected cells in order to kill the infected cell. By damaging the integrity of cell membranes, the contents are then available for destruction. Cytotoxic T-cells also elicit a form of programmed cell death called apoptosis, whereby infected cells are "told" to commit suicide. This process is common in viruses such as HIV. Potent cytokines, gamma-interferon and tumor necrosis factor are also released to inhibit viral replication and bring other immune warriors such as macrophages to destroy the cell. This mechanism has dangerous repercussions in certain viral infections. Infections that are rapid and excessive, as is found in the Ebola virus, may cause a wave of destruction to multiple organs or systems in the body, ultimately causing death.

No Response Can Be Better

While on one hand an aggressive immune response to infection may cause destruction of the host, other defense mechanisms to invaders may be ineffective and allow viruses to live undetected within cells for months or even years. Minor damage to the host may occur, but if the immune system does not see the invader as a threat it can allow it to continue unchecked. This is true for the hepatitis A virus, which poses little danger to healthy individuals. Also, chronic carriers of hepatitis B generally suffer liver damage even though the virus is relatively harmless. Immunologists believe that the liver damage that results in the case of hepatitis B is caused by the cell-destroying action of cytotoxic T-cells. While eradicating the virus, these cells damage liver tissue.

On the other hand, the immune system may allow cells harboring viruses to survive in order to ensure that the immune response does not kill too many cells and cause injury to the host. This adaptation, featured by a lack of a responsive immune attack, will protect the host in the long run, especially if the immune system is unable to control the virus without causing irreparable harm to the body's tissues. This protective feature is a positive adaptation as long as the invader does not lead to serious tissue abnormalities or death.

Viruses, bacteria and parasites pose constant challenges to the immune system. By their nature they are constantly mutating and evolving in order to avoid detection. Viruses have subverted the cell's machinery in order to ensure its reproduction and survival. In certain pathogenic infections, the microorganism will use the cell's own factors to assist in the replication of the invader. This is the mechanism that HIV uses to ensure its survival.

HIV INFECTION

Since the discovery of the acquired immunodeficiency syndrome (AIDS) in 1980, millions of dollars of research have gone into the search for an effective cure and vaccine. After almost two decades of research, it is now clear that AIDS is a serious threat to human health and life. Although other infectious diseases such as malaria kill more people than AIDS, the lack of effective vaccines and treatments makes AIDS an especially alarming disease. No other virus in history has received such extensive study.

Many strains of HIV exist and some are more deadly than others. In West Africa, HIV-2 is common, and produces a weaker disease than HIV-1, which is deadly. Researchers also believe that some forms of HIV may not be dangerous to our health at all. There are cases of men infected with HIV for more than 15 years without ever showing any symptoms of AIDS.

Opinions on the cause of AIDS vary, but HIV infection is currently believed to be the source of the disease. The dominant feature of the syndrome is the deficiency of circulating helper T-cells. Scientists feel that HIV alone will cause serious immune dysfunction without the help of other viruses. Yet people who are immune compromised, of course, are more susceptible to a multitude of infectious states. Often it is those infections that hasten death in an HIV-infected individual.

The Anatomy of HIV

Unlike other viruses of the common cold, influenza or hepatitis, HIV reproduces itself inside the cells of the immune system. It is a retrovirus that hijacks helper T-cells and dominates the cell's genetic makeup. HIV is able to change its nature from month to month, making it very difficult to destroy or produce an effective vaccine. The flu virus is similar in its ability to mutate quickly, hence the reason for different vaccines for the many flu strains each year.

HIV's principal target cells are helper T-cells. This is a smart move on the part of the virus because helper T-cells activate the other components of the immune system. They act like generals, telling cytotoxic T-cells to attack virus-infected cells and B-cells to produce antibodies. In the case of HIV-infected helper T-cells, these commands are subverted and the virus is left to thrive.

HIV is transmitted through blood and body fluids, including blood, semen, vaginal secretions, tears, urine, saliva and breast milk. Upon infection, the immune system mounts a serious defensive. In some cases it is believed that the immune response is powerful enough to eradicate the virus. Most often, however, by the time B-cells produce antibodies, infection is complete and permanent. After the cells are infected, most people develop acute flu-like symptoms: fever, skin rashes, general weakness and muscle aches, and enlarged lymph glands of the groin, neck and under the arms similar to glandular fever. The liver and spleen may also become enlarged. These symptoms may last approximately two weeks and then disappear, but during this time transmission of the disease to others is easy. After this initial infection, it may take up to 12 months before a person will test positive for HIV antibodies and they will still feel quite well. After several years, opportunistic infections and cancers may start appearing.

HIV and AIDS Statistics

- Health Canada reports the number of AIDS cases to date to be approximately 20,000.

- It is estimated that 36,000 to 42,000 Canadians are living with HIV.

- Worldwide, it is estimated that 30 million people are infected with HIV/AIDS.

- Every day, 16,000 people become infected with HIV.

- In 1997, 2.3 million people died of AIDS; 50 percent of those deaths were women.

- More than 1 million children are now living with HIV; 2.7 million children have already died from the disease.

- Contrary to public perception, heterosexual, not homosexual, sex is the major route of transmission.

AIDS Diagnosis

Healthy individuals normally have T-cell counts between 800 to 1,200 per cubic millimeter. When this count drops to approximately 200 or less, along with the presence of an opportunistic infection such as pneumocystis carinii pneumonia, Kaposi's sarcoma, demential or lymphoid involvement and other diseases, full-blown AIDS is the diagnosis. It may take a decade or more for full-blown AIDS to develop after the initial infection with HIV and, as discussed above, some of those infected in the discovery years of the disease have yet to acquire symptoms.

Many theories suggest reasons for the decline in T-cell counts. Cytotoxic T-cells are an important line of defense against viruses that live inside cells and as a result they are involved in the destruction of infected helper T-cells. This is a double-edged response, as destruction of HIV-infected cells also causes immune deficiency. Programmed cell death, apoptosis, also occurs, although the mechanism is not clearly understood. Both mechanisms lead to a decline in helper T-cell counts. Moreover, HIV-infected people are found to have high levels of interleukin-6, which promotes inflammation and tissue destruction.

HIV and Balance between T_H1 and T_H2 Cells

HIV infection causes a decline in the ability of T_H1 cells to produce protective interleukin-2. In the early nineties it was proposed that the immune dysfunction caused by HIV may be due to an imbalance of T_H1 to T_H2 cells. Researchers have discovered that persons just infected with HIV are predominantly T_H1, and in as little as a few years this changes to a T_H2 dominance. It is believed that those HIV-infected individuals who remain symptom free after infection have higher T_H1 cells. In *Basic and Clinical Immunology* the authors Mark Peakman and Diego Vergani state that, "The search is on for therapies that may selectively enhance T_H1 and dampen T_H2 responses." Synthetic interleukin-2 has been tried, but failed as a method to selectively promote T_H1.

Sterinol Effective at Halting Helper T-Cell Decline

Sterinol does exactly what Peakman and Vergani were stating. It "selectively enhances T_H1" and the production of interleukin-2. Patrick Bouic and his research team at Stellenbosch University, have confirmed this theory in an open-labeled study with a small control group with 323 HIV-infected patients. The study began in 1993 and the patients, diagnosed HIV-positive, were followed for more than five years. Blood parameters including helper T-cell determination, degree of apoptosis (programmed cell death), serum cytokine (measurement of the pro-inflammatory interleukin-6, which was shown to activate viral replication in infected cells) and plasma (plasma is the fluid part of the blood, lymph or human milk; viral is the virus; and load means the total number of cells infected) RNA viral load were determined.

The trial comprised two groups of subjects: one that received Sterinol and a control group, all monitored at Tygerberg Hospital's infectious disease clinic. Results from this study showed that helper T-cells did not drop in the Sterinol treatment group, compared to the control group. At the six-month point in the trial, members of the control group were offered the Sterinol treatment because their helper T-cells were dropping at the expected rate in HIV infection, and there was a risk of death. Researchers felt that it was unethical to allow these people to die, knowing that the Sterinol group did not exhibit the same downward spiral of helper T-cell decline. As well, apoptosis, which is proposed as a reason for the excessive helper T-cell loss in HIV-infected individuals, did not show a statistically significant decline; the degree of cell death in the blood of the subjects taking Sterinol showed a slight decline.

Interleukin-6, the pro-inflammatory cytokine that is implicated in the virus's ability to replicate, decreased significantly in the Sterinol group. Many researchers recommend antioxidants to help inhibit interleukin-6—another reason to supplement with the super-immune nutrients discussed in chapter 3.

Sterols and sterolins were not found to have antiviral activity in humans, but it is thought that long-term use may change this. Unfortunately, viral loads were not conducted on all patients since commercial tests were not available until late in the study. However, in those who were tested, a slow decline in viral load was noticed over a 6-9 month period, but this decrease is not as dramatic as that induced by current antivirals.

On a visit to South Africa, Professor Luc Montagnier, the man who discovered the HI virus, discussed with Bouic's research team the value of sterols and sterolins in the therapy for HIV-infected people as an effective, affordable, non-toxic immune modulator to be used in conjunction with antivirals. In most of the world, the cost of HIV/AIDS treatments are prohibitive, especially in Africa, where patients do not have the money for drugs and the state does not provide free health care. Essentially, if you are diagnosed with HIV and cannot afford treatment, you will die.

To date, Bouic's research indicates that helper T-cells are stabilized with a decrease in serum pro-inflammatory interleukin-6. We are currently awaiting the results of a new trial, to be initiated under the auspices of Professor Montagnier in Paris, whereby the patients will be treated with sterols and sterolins together with lower doses of antivirals.

The importance of Sterinol in the treatment of HIV/AIDS cannot be understated. It should be the basis that all other adjuncts are added to. Even current antivirals do not offer an effective method to ensure helper T-cell decline is stopped. Sterinol will ensure that those infected with the virus will be able to live with the virus.

Living with the AIDS Virus

AIDS is a highly complex disease, and in no way do we wish to deny that. If you are currently taking the AIDS cocktail of antivirals, do not stop unless your health care professional recommends it. The suggestions we make here should be used as adjuvants. We want you to understand that the following research is provided to help you or someone you love who is infected with HIV to live a long and healthy life.

Currently, there is no cure for AIDS and our focus should be on providing the immune system with adequate tools to ensure the longest life possible with the least symptoms. The suggestions discussed below should be incorporated into a treatment protocol, along with the immune system cure diet. We recommend that those infected with HIV and AIDS adopt the lifestyle suggestions made earlier, especially those that pertain to emotional status (see chapter 6). Remember, your mental and emotional state play a role in immunity—negative and positive.

More Natural Therapies

DHEA and HIV Infection

The progression of HIV to full-blown AIDS is affected by complex changes in the production of adrenal steroids, specifically cortisol and dehydroepiandrosterone (DHEA). Elevated cortisol levels are seen in many diseases of the immune system, with a corresponding decline in protective DHEA levels. This is especially true in persons with HIV, in whom dehydroepiandrosterone sulfate (DHEAS) and its derivative, DHEA, antagonists of cortisol, are low. As well, the shift from T_H1-dominant helper cells to T_H2 helper cells is encouraged by the increase in cortisol and the reduction of DHEA. As discussed above, when T_H1 helper cells are suppressed and T_H2 is in excess, a cascade of immune-related problems occurs; for example, cancer is left to flourish, inflammation occurs and autoimmune diseases run rampant. It has also been found that an increase in the production of cortisol may be related to the rapid cell death in helper T-cells in HIV-infected persons. It is believed that by balancing the cortisol-to-DHEA ratio, a reduction in T_H2 helper cell factors will occur. This will then allow the good T_H1 immune factors to be released—a process that will balance the immune system.

Sterols and Sterolins Increase DHEA

Sterols and sterolins are precursors to pregnenolone and then DHEA. They also cause a dominance in T_H1 cells and a subsequent reduction in cortisol levels. A daily dosage of 6 capsules for one week, taken on an empty stomach with a maintenance dose of 3 capsules per day thereafter will help keep the cortisol-to-DHEA ratio in check. Supplementation with Sterinol will increase DHEA levels to the individual's optimal personal level over the long term (each person's level will be specific to them).

DHEA can also be supplemented directly. A DHEA blood test should be performed in order to determine the correct dosage. Depending on the age of the person and their disease state, dosages vary dramatically.

Vitamin C for HIV

Drs. Robert Cathcart, Frederick Klenner, Linus Pauling and Ian Brighthope have used vitamin C to treat viral conditions, with amazing benefits. Intravenous and oral vitamin C supplementation (see chapter 3) are used by both Cathcart and Brighthope to treat HIV-infected individuals. Buffered vitamin C in the form of mineral ascorbates should be taken orally to bowel tolerance to slow replication of the HI virus. Intravenous vitamin C treatment is administered by your health care professional. Sodium ascorbate, at 60 to 150 g per day, have been administered intravenously with dramatic results. Vitamin C works by stimulating the immune system to operate more efficiently while it stimulates enzymes necessary for detoxification of chemicals and other environmental pollutants. It also has a powerful antifungal, antiparasitic, antibacterial and antiviral action, all necessary for the treatment of secondary infections in HIV-infected individuals. (See chapter 3 for more information on vitamin C; and read *The AIDS Fighters* by Ian Brighthope for detailed information on HIV and IV infusions of vitamin C.)

ABCs OF HEPATITIS

Hepatitis is a liver disease caused by the viruses hepatitis A, hepatitis B and hepatitis C. Each virus differs in the symptoms that develop, in the route of transmission and in the severity and long-term consequences.

Hepatitis A

The virus that causes hepatitis A lives in human feces and is passed on to unsuspecting recipients through contaminated food and water. It is the most common of the three viruses. Members of the same household or those in close contact with an infected individual are most susceptible. Poor hygiene and sanitation are the reason for the widespread transmission of hepatitis A. Restaurants are often the source of an outbreak of hepatitis A. Day-care centers where workers do not wash their hands after changing soiled diapers are also a common source of the disease. Fruits and vegetables can also be a source of hepatitis A when water that is contaminated is used for irrigation.

The virus will survive in raw or undercooked food, especially in shellfish that has come from waters contaminated with raw sewage. It is surprising that in technology-driven North America, waters could be the home to raw sewage, but many communities do not have sewage treatment plants.

Symptoms of hepatitis A, which can last from several weeks to months in more severe cases, include fever, nausea, vomiting, fatigue, diarrhea, appetite loss, elevated liver enzymes and yellowing of the skin and whites of the eyes—jaundice, caused by increased bilirubin in the blood. Bilirubin is a reddish-yellow substance that naturally occurs in bile, blood, urine and gallstones. Yellow skin and increased bilirubin counts both occur for several weeks. Hepatitis A is rarely fatal, although the elderly and those with compromised immune systems are at risk. Unlike hepatitis B and C, the disease does not cause long-term liver damage, and once infected you are immune from the virus a second time around.

Hepatitis B

Unprotected sex is the most common method of transmission of the virus that causes hepatitis B, although blood can also be a source. Unlike hepatitis A, the disease is not spread by contaminated food. It can also be spread from an infected mother to her newborn during the birth process. Without treatment, these babies become high risk for long-term chronic hepatitis B. Sharp instruments such as dental tools, tattoo needles, body piercing implements, razors and toothbrushes can be carriers of the virus.

Flu-like symptoms, dark urine, jaundice and profound fatigue are some of the symptoms of hepatitis B. Each year, 222,000 North Americans contract hepatitis B. Most of those people are able to clear the virus from their body without any long-term consequences. The other small percentage develop chronic hepatitis because their immune system is unable to eradicate the virus.

Liver damage in the form of cirrhosis or liver cancer can result from chronic hepatitis. Infected individuals are also able to transmit the virus to those with whom they have unprotected intimate contact. Hepatitis B kills approximately 6,000 people annually in Canada and the United States.

Hepatitis C

Hepatitis C is now seen in epidemic proportions. In Canada, liver specialists are overwhelmed as they struggle to deal with an increase in hepatitis C cases. There are an estimated 275,000 hepatitis C patients, most as a result of tainted blood transfusions prior to 1992. In the United States, more than 4 million people suffer from chronic hepatitis C, and it is the leading cause for liver transplants.

The disease is spread through the transmission of blood and body fluids, but unprotected sex is not the main route of infection. Intravenous drug users, health care workers, lab technicians and emergency or ambulance workers are all at high risk of contracting hepatitis C. Moreover, there was no blood test to screen for hepatitis C until 1992, and as a result, many people were infected with tainted blood through blood transfusions.

Flu-like symptoms may or may not be present. Some people have no symptoms at all and yet harbor the virus. Unlike hepatitis A and B, hepatitis C almost always leads to chronic disease. Over 85 percent develop chronic hepatitis as the virus slowly and insidiously destroys the liver, with 5 percent developing liver cancer.

Medical Therapies for Hepatitis

What all three viruses have in common is the lack of effective medical therapies to treat them. Vaccines for hepatitis A and B are available to prevent infection. So far, there is no vaccine for hepatitis C. Current drug therapies are ineffective and fraught with serious side effects. Alpha-interferon is used with minimal success to treat hepatitis B and C, with only 35 percent of cases gaining any benefit, and hair loss, severe nausea and depression as side effects of treatment. A new treatment combining the antiviral drug Ribavirin with alpha-interferon eliminates the virus in 45 percent of cases but comes with a hefty price tag and the risk of birth defects to the developing fetus, if you happen to be pregnant when you take the treatment.

Sterols and Sterolins for Hepatitis

The damage that results from the hepatitis virus is a result of the immune system attacking liver cells while trying to destroy the virus. Sterols and sterolins stop this destruction by reducing the effects of T_H2 helper cells and their cytokine, interleukin-6, while stimulating T_H1 cells to proliferate, allowing for a liver tissue protective effect. We recommend a dose of 6 capsules each day for seven days, then 3 capsules per day thereafter. Rapid return of liver enzymes to normal parameters is seen in patients supplementing with Sterinol.

Hepatitis C is a serious viral condition whereby the immune system exacerbates the problem while trying to destroy the virus. Conventional treatments are less than satisfactory and side effects from the drugs used to treat the disease are terrible; for example, severe hair loss, depression and nausea. Considering that those who suffer from chronic hepatitis C have a high risk for liver cancer and/or the need for liver transplantation, Sterinol is an effective method to control the immune system while eradicating the virus. If you have already had a liver transplant, however, Sterinol is contraindicated.

A PHYSICIAN'S RESPONSE TO STERINOL

Dr. Stewart Gibson treated a 70-year-old patient with chronic active hepatitis C that was the result of a blood transfusion four years earlier. The patient had a white cell count of .9 and her platelets were lower than 42. Dr. Gibson initiated a course of Intron A at 3 million units three times a week and increased this dose to 10 million units two times a week, which was the maximum the patient could tolerate. The patient continued this regimen for two months, with no change in her blood parameters. At this point the doctor added Legalon 70, 1 tablet three times a day, in addition to the Intron A. After several months, the Intron A was stopped. Then sterols and sterolins were added, 1 capsule three times a day for several months. At this point, another liver function test was performed and the results were phenomenal. The patient was still taking the Legalon, but she was given this when the Intron A was used without any change in liver function. Dr. Gibson deduced that due to the Sterinol, the viral insult to his patient's liver had been inhibited. Her platelet count rose to 65 and she no longer had extensive reddish-purple spots on her forearms and legs. Although this is "just" an anecdotal case, only 30 percent of hepatitis C patients improve on Intron A. Dr. Gibson believes that the difference in his patient's liver function is due to Sterinol.

Adopt the nutritional recommendations for infectious diseases and include milk thistle or silymarin to help detoxify and strengthen the liver. Take 100 to 200 mg three times a day until your symptoms are alleviated.

Dr. Robert Cathcart and others have used intravenous vitamin C to wipe out the hepatitis C virus. A dosage of 50 to 100 grams, delivered intravenously, generally eradicates acute hepatitis within 2 to 4 days and jaundice within 1 week. Talk to your medical practitioner for IV vitamin C therapy.

TUBERCULOSIS

Tuberculosis is an infection caused by the bacterium mycobacterium tuberculosis (TB). The infection can either be short-lived or chronic, affecting the lungs or other body sites. Early symptoms of TB include a morning cough and fever, flu-like aches and pains, as well as chest pain, labored breathing, coughing up blood, poor appetite, severe weight loss and night sweats. In severe cases, dangerous complications can arise, causing death.

In North America, TB causes approximately 2,000 deaths annually. Until recently, it was believed that TB was under control in the United States and Canada. Due to transcontinental air travel, however, the disease has had a resurgence. TB is transmitted through contact with airborne infected sputum secreted from a coughing individual. People with compromised immune systems are more vulnerable to this bacterium, such as HIV-infected persons, those with diabetes and those who are malnourished.

Corticosteroids used in the treatment of autoimmune diseases such as rheumatoid arthritis cause immune suppression and allow diseases such as TB easy access.

Treatment for tuberculosis includes powerful antibacterial drugs which should be used in combination with the immune-boosting diet suggested in this book and Sterinol.

Sterols and Sterolin: TB Research

The treatment of tuberculosis has been so refined that 95 percent of patients who comply with the therapy can be successfully treated with a six-month regimen of a combination of the drugs mentioned above. Despite this, close to 25 percent of tuberculosis patients in developing countries may fail to complete their therapy, leading to high relapse rates and the danger of contracting drug-resistant tuberculosis.

While undergoing therapy, many TB patients experience severe weight loss, which in itself carries health risks. In view of the considerable deficiencies of current tuberculosis regimens, researchers in South Africa examined the effect of sterols and sterolins in pulmonary tuberculosis patients.

Patrick Bouic and his team of researchers conducted a study at DP Marais Tuberculosis Hospital of the South African National Tuberculosis Association in Cape Town where they looked at the adjuvant effects of Sterinol in the treatment of pulmonary tuberculosis. This area of South Africa has a particularly high incidence of tuberculosis; in 1993, the rate was over 500 for every 100,000 people. Twenty-three patients were included in the treatment group to receive Sterinol, along with a combination of the standard tuberculosis drugs Isoniazid, Rifampicin and Pyrazinamide. Subjects were confirmed for their TB by sputum smear microscopy for mycobacterium tuberculosis and then randomized to receive either Sterinol or placebo. The allocation of the patients to the different treatment groups was unknown to those conducting the trial. Patients were evaluated on admission and thereafter monthly with regard to weight gain, by X ray, full blood count, white cell count, sputum culture and liver function tests. Patients participated in the study for a minimum of four months. Patients who had drug-resistant tuberculosis were excluded from the analysis.

Of the 23 patients who received sterols and sterolins, 4 were subsequently excluded, 1 died after three months of treatment, 1 was found to have multi-drug-resistant (to both Rifampicin and Isoniazid) tuberculosis, 1 was HIV-positive and 1 patient abandoned treatment after a month. Eighteen patients remained in the placebo group. At the end of the study, the most dramatic feature of the sterol and sterolin group was that of weight gain. Weight loss is a serious symptom of tuberculosis; many health complications arise as a result. In the sterol and sterolin–treated group, there was a significant rise in weight. There was also a significant normalization of blood parameters and an increase in lymphocytes and eosinophils (white blood cells) as was expected from past research using sterols and sterolins.

All people with infectious diseases should take 2 capsules of Sterinol three times a day for one week, and 1 capsule three times a day for maintenance.

ANTIBIOTIC-RESISTANT BACTERIA

Over the last several years certain strains of bacteria have become resistant to antibiotic therapies. For example, Vancomycin is the antibiotic that carried the most clout and now bacteria have devised a method to resist it. Bacterial species including enterococcus faecalis, mycobacterium tuberculosis and Pseudomonas aeruginosa have learned how to evade treatment by almost 100 drugs. Until recently, diseases such as TB were thought to be under control, and we mistakenly believed that antibiotics were effectively dealing with all bacteria. The reality is, we no longer have effective treatments for common bacteria. And we must understand that we are mostly at fault for this.

Overuse of antibiotics is the main reason for bacteria becoming resistant to these drugs. More than 50 million pounds of antibiotics are produced annually in North America. People insist on antibiotics for viral diseases, upon which an antibiotic has absolutely no effect. In their quest to keep patients happy, many physicians continue to supply the required prescriptions. If your doctor suspects a bacterial infection for which antibiotics need to be prescribed, simple tests can confirm the presence of the bacteria before prescribing antibiotic treatment. Antibiotics should be viewed as serious medications and only prescribed as a last resort. Ear infections, common in children, is one example where antibiotic therapy rarely works to eliminate the problem, and several prescriptions may be prescribed to deal with the recurrent symptoms. Physicians are now being trained to treat common childhood infections cautiously with antibiotics.

Second, misuse of antibiotics, which includes not completing a course of therapy, has allowed bacteria the opportunity to mutate and become resistant to future treatment. Moreover, flushing leftover antibiotics down the drain or allowing them to go to the landfill have polluted the environment. Worse yet is saving the antibiotic to treat undiagnosed illnesses at a later date. Creams, ointments and soaps are now loaded with antibacterial agents; even these should be used cautiously, as bacteria may incorporate these into their genetic makeup, allowing resistance to develop.

Domestic animals are fed large quantities of antibiotics to keep them healthy in their unnatural environments. We then eat these antibiotics when we consume the animal product. Beef, poultry and farm-grown fish are laden with antibiotic residues. Farmers must search for safer ways to encourage animal growth and health.

Good hygiene, especially washing your hands often, is the most effective method of controlling the spread of bacteria. Let's not believe that we will always have an antibiotic that works for every bacteria. It may well be that one day we won't, and we will have to rely entirely on our immune system to battle the bacteria.

CHRONIC FATIGUE SYNDROME

Chronic fatigue syndrome (CFS) is an immune system disease that affects millions of North Americans. Many CFS sufferers cannot continue to work, some are bedridden and others can only work part-time. Chronic fatigue syndrome produces a profound fatigue state including weakness, swollen glands, fever, problems with balance, brain lesions, depression and a severe lack of energy, lasting up to several years in serious cases. Women account for the majority of those affected by the disorder.

So diverse and transient are the symptoms of chronic fatigue that it has been maligned and misdiagnosed as depression and other mental illness. Some sufferers have been labeled as hypochondriacs for their many visits to endless numbers of physicians and specialists. To put an end to the difficulty in diagnosing CFS, the Centers for Disease Control, Atlanta, Georgia, developed criteria to be used in evaluating this unusual syndrome. The protocol states that "onset of debilitating fatigue must persist in a steady or recurring state for at least six months and halt normal daily activities over fifty percent of the time." Low-grade fever, sore throat, chills, muscle and joint aches and weakness, sleep problems, mental confusion and emotional imbalance are also included in the criteria.

Other serious diseases such as rheumatoid arthritis, multiple sclerosis and lupus also predominantly affect women. Some researchers believe that viruses may be at the root of these disease states, and many feel that chronic fatigue may also be the result of viral infections. It is thought that Epstein Barr virus (EBV), cytomegalovirus, herpes simplex virus, both oral and genital and herpes type-6 virus may be the cause of CFS and the subsequent dysfunction of the immune system. We know that viruses have the ability to alter normal immune function in order to maintain their survival and even subvert normal attack mechanisms so that they can lie dormant for years, even decades. It is thought that these dormant viruses are allowed to replicate when the immune system stops functioning properly, encouraging the syndrome of chronic fatigue.

We learned earlier that emotions and nutritional status are important factors in whether the immune system is able to fight off invaders. Once depressed, the body's defense mechanisms are unable to inhibit parasitic, yeast, fungal, viral and bacterial infections. Parasites are thought to play a major role in the development of CFS. Their ability to weaken the body has serious long-term health implications. Over and over we have discussed how microorganisms that used to be efficiently handled by our immune systems are now wreaking havoc with our health. It is imperative that we realize this and take action to ensure our survival. Eliminate toxins as much as possible, feed your body what it needs both nutritionally and spiritually—for your health's sake.

Immune Problems and CFS

Persons with CFS have down-regulated antibody levels and few natural killer cells. They also release less of the good cytokines gamma-interferon and interleukin-2, as well as tumor necrosis factor alpha. When natural killer cells are low, parasites and viruses can gain hold and flourish. Cancer cells are also able to freely proliferate in the absence of natural killer cells.

People with CFS have elevated helper T-cell to suppressor T-cell ratios and elevated B-cells and autoantibodies in the blood. High histamine is another immune symptom recognized in CFS patients that causes diarrhea and allergic symptoms. Over 65 percent of CFS sufferers have symptoms of allergies. CFS individuals also have low blood levels of the immune-regulating hormone DHEA and higher than average levels of cortisol.

Treatments that are most effective at eliminating the syndrome should be based on putting the immune system back into a state of balance whereby it can fight off common invaders that have a powerful role in the progression of all diseases.

Sterols and Sterolins for CFS

Sterols and sterolins enhance the activity of the T-cells by inducing the synthesis of the immune-regulatory cytokines interleukin-2 and gamma-interferon while decreasing the inflammation-causing cytokine interleukin-4. This ultimately leads to the control of allergic conditions, autoimmune processes and the ability of the immune response to deal with latent viruses, bacteria or parasites. As discussed earlier, one of the most striking benefits to the immune system from the inclusion of sterols and sterolins is the enhancement of natural killer cell activity, the body's most powerful line of defense against cancer cells and microorganisms.

We also know that sterols and sterolins are effective at enhancing DHEA levels, causing a decrease in the stress hormone cortisol. This is also seen in persons with HIV, rheumatoid arthritis and systemic lupus erythematosus.

We recommend a dosage of 6 capsules per day for the first week then 3 capsules per day thereafter for a balanced immune system.

Other Immune Nutrients for CFS

Adopt the protocol for infectious disease at the end of this chapter and add the following specific nutrients for chronic fatigue.

Coenzyme Q_{10} was discussed in chapter 3, yet it needs special attention for those with impaired cellular and natural immunity as seen in CFS sufferers. The powerful antioxidant is especially important during viral infections since CoQ_{10} levels in white blood cells fall rapidly as the cell's requirements for this super-immune nutrient increase in order to fight off invaders. CoQ_{10} stimulates the immune system to kill bacteria and increase antibody response. It also maximizes the eating and digesting ability of macrophages, allowing them to destroy bacteria, viruses and parasites effectively. Serum IgG levels have also been shown to increase with very small doses (60 mg) of CoQ_{10}. It is also known to enhance natural killer cell activity and inhibit metastasis of tumors.

Most important for CFS sufferers is CoQ_{10}'s ability to increase adenosine tri-phosphate (ATP) production. ATP is needed to provide sufficient energy to the body. Without adequate ATP, we feel tired and experience muscle weakness and impaired immunity. Cells of the immune system, muscles and heart have a high affinity for CoQ_{10}, and when supplies are inadequate, disease states settle in.

A dosage of 320 mg per day of CoQ_{10} should be supplemented to ensure that appropriate levels are available to immune cells during infection. CoQ_{10} is one of the safest nutrients available, but if you are currently taking digitalis, beta-blockers or ACE inhibitors, your prescription drug dose will need to be lowered once you start it.

Certain vitamins and minerals have powerful effects on the immune system. To summarize from chapter 3, the following should be supplemented daily: quercetin, reduced L-glutathione, CoQ_{10}, magnesium, B complex, zinc, vitamins A and E and selenium. Moreover, herbs including St. John's wort, echinacea, shiitake mushroom, garlic and licorice root are well known for their antiviral, antibacterial and anticancer properties. They are important immune stimulants. Remember the importance of the superstar phytonutrient sterols and sterolins, as they are important immune modulators that balance the immune system, allowing it to operate as it was designed to do.

Alcohol, cigarettes and prescription drugs are all immunotoxins that should be eliminated when an infectious disease sets in, especially hepatitis. All three are detoxified by the liver and any added burden to this major organ will impede healing.

SUGGESTED SUPPLEMENT PROGRAM FOR INFECTIOUS MICROORGANISMS

Adopt the immune system cure diet, obtain adequate rest, think positively, perform gentle exercises and love and laugh at life's challenges.

We recommend 6 capsules of Sterinol per day for 1 week, and 3 capsules per day thereafter. If you only take one supplement, take this one.

Supplemental Nutrients for Infections

Vitamin C orally to bowel tolerance	intravenous infusions 50 g daily for two weeks
Vitamin A	micellized vitamin A, 100,000 IU, one dropperful on the first day; 20,000 IU or 4 drops daily for maintenance
Vitamin E	1,200 IU per day; micellized vitamin E, 1 ml twice daily, or natural vitamin E with mixed tocopherols 3, 400 IU capsules
Selenium	Selenomethionine, 200 mcg daily
High-potency B complex	2 capsules twice daily
Zinc citrate	60 mg daily
Magnesium glycinate	100 mg twice daily
Weleda iscador (mistletoe) injections	1.0 ml injected subcutaneously
Lactobacillus acidophilus powder	2 teaspoons daily
Garlic capsules	3 capsules daily
Lipoic Acid	500 mg twice daily
Udo's Choice Oil or Omega Balance	2 tablespoons daily with food
Reduced L-glutathione	150 mg twice daily
Licorice root extract	5 ml twice daily
Digestive enzymes at each meal	2 capsules

STRESS, EXERCISE AND IMMUNITY

O Excellent, I love long life better than figs.

—William Shakespeare

Excessive stress, either physical or mental, has a detrimental effect on the optimal functioning of the immune system. It is like the card that finally tips the balance on the house of cards, bringing everything crashing down. An immune system that is in top operating order will only be minimally affected by small stressors, yet that same system can be toppled by a big stressor such as the death of a loved one. Conversely, even small stressors can be too much for a weakened immune system.

What causes our immune system to become unbalanced, deficient and hyperstimulated? Simply stated, most of the health problems of the late 20th century are attributable to two things: stress and nutrition. According to many physicians, stress has surpassed the cold virus as the most common health problem in North America. Living with the type of stress that does not go away or just feeling as if you can't get out from under stress is enough to cause disease. The effort to succeed, to compete, to have more and do more have all contributed to many of our health problems.

Although we may not be aware of them, there are many types of stressors that affect us daily: noise, crowded cities, our polluted environment, a lack of exposure to the sun, driving, crime, racism, pathogens, a lack of joy in our lives, abuse, school, work, negative emotions, loneliness and much more. When these stressors accumulate, they wreak havoc with our immune system and, ultimately, allow viruses, bacteria and cancer cells to take hold and reproduce, causing mayhem with our health.

Scientists now confirm that our response to stressors has a profound effect on the body's ability to protect itself from everyday infections and life-threatening illness such as cancer. In *The Stress of Life*, Dr. Hans Selye wrote, "If a microbe is in or around us all the time and yet causes no disease until we are exposed to stress, what is the cause of the illness, the microbe or the stress?" Dr. Selye believed that both played a role in the development of disease. A serious illness is often preceded by a major life stressor such as a death, loss of a job, illness of a loved one, even moving to a new location. Will antibiotics be truly effective if the source of the stress is not removed, and will we take longer to recover as a result? We know that every time we are exposed to a bacteria or virus, we do not contract an infection. A lower immune resistance caused by excessive stress, poor nutrition and toxins in the environment are the pendulum that swings toward illness.

STRESS AND DISEASE

You will often hear people tell the story of a friend who just had a heart attack or was diagnosed with cancer. "He was so healthy," they say. "We just can't understand how he could have contracted it," they add. They go on to report that he was careful about his diet, jogged 3 miles five days a week and looked great. Well, exercise and diet alone cannot prevent disease. As discussed in chapter 6, the mind plays a major role in ensuring that we have maximum immunity. Stress plays the most powerful role. Yes, you can give your body more B vitamins and magnesium, and these will replenish some of the nutrients lost during stressful times. You can eat better to support the body. But unless you deal with the stressors in your life, you are only putting a Band-Aid on your health problems.

Stress is the number-one universal risk factor for major disease development. Good physicians will ask their patients about the stress they confront in their lives and how they deal with it. Stress is the biggest factor in the development of heart disease and cancer. There are people with normal blood parameters for heart disease that are at high risk for heart attack because they deal with stress poorly or just have too much stress in their lives. One common factor among 20,000 women studied after they had been diagnosed with breast cancer was that they felt trapped in their lives, trapped in their marriages and saw no way to break free. The important factor here was not that they were trapped but that they *felt* trapped.

Heart attacks are more common on Monday morning than at any other time. Researchers believe it is a response to returning to a job that one hates or feels trapped in. If you hate your job, find a new one. Make a concerted effort to actively find a solution to this problem. The stress of having to go to a job in which you are unhappy or unfulfilled is devastating to certain organs, especially the heart. Your life may depend on changing your job. The good news is that stress is one factor in your life that you actually can change.

ONE PERSON'S STRESS IS ANOTHER'S PLAY

Stress means different things to different people. You may find lecturing fun, while for someone else it is an extremely stress-provoking event. Picture two lecturers waiting outside a packed auditorium for their presentations to begin. One is excited and looking forward to sharing knowledge with the people inside. Her heart rate is up slightly, but this gives her an edge and allows memory recall to be a little sharper. The other lecturer has visited the bathroom three times with stress-induced diarrhea and a nagging urge to urinate. His heart rate has increased so much he hears it beating in his ears, and on top of that, he can't remember anything he is supposed to say. These two people are experiencing very different responses to the same stimulus: one feels positive anticipation; the other fear and apprehension. Stress is determined by our response to situations and this means that it is very difficult to define.

Physiologically, the body has developed mechanisms to protect it from the damaging effects of stress. However, if stress is relentless or extreme, these same mechanisms can become harmful. The flight-or-fight response is one way the body deals with extreme situations of stress. Upon realizing we are in danger, the brain sounds an alarm, telling our adrenal glands to secrete adrenaline and cortisol, which mobilizes the body to fight or run away and find protection. Most of us have heard the story of the bystander who picks up the car under which a child was trapped. Our fight response is the source of this amazing show of superhuman strength.

This response is supposed to be a short-lived reaction, yet today most of us are in and out of this state continually due to such stressors as pressures at work, driving in rush-hour traffic and not having enough time and too much to do. Prolonged physical, psychological and social stressors cause our immune system to become imbalanced. As a result, our adrenal glands become exhausted from continually having to produce regulatory factors and we experience weakened body systems, especially the cardiovascular, immune and endocrine systems. Exhausted adrenals shrink in a similar way to the shrinking of the thymus gland (see chapter 2), and with this side effect the factors that are secreted decline.

The adrenal glands also produce DHEA, the superpowered hormone. When the adrenals become exhausted, conditions of immune dysfunction appear, including allergies, autoimmune disorders, colds and flu, chronic infections, irritable bowel syndrome, headaches and cancer. Feeling fatigued and stressed-out are common complaints that result from exhausted adrenals.

EVERYTHING IS UNDER CONTROL

An optimistic outlook on the stressors you confront in life is immune-system protective. People who have learned effective coping mechanisms and who work to find solutions to their problems not only feel better but do not waste energy on the things they can't change. Setting realistic goals, developing strong self-esteem and seeking knowledge are all methods of stress management.

Tense and Relax Technique

One stress reduction method taught to first-year university psychology students is a tense-and-relax technique. Start with the muscles of your face and neck and work your way down the body until you reach your toes. Tense the muscles of your face for two full seconds then release and relax. Remember to inhale deeply when you tense your muscles and exhale deeply when you release them. Next, contract your neck and shoulder muscles and then release. Continue working your way down the body and be aware of all the tension you are letting go through this process. You may need to repeat the process 2 or 3 times to completely de-stress your muscles.

Protect your body by eliminating as much stress as possible, and learn how to cope with what you can't get rid of. Adopt some of the stress management techniques mentioned in chapter 6, and add the nutrients we mention here, specifically designed to treat stress-induced disease states, to your super-immune nutrient program.

FRIENDS AND FAMILY OFFER COMFORT

We can not say enough about the power of supportive social networks, good friends, family, church and social groups to help us work out stress. People who have active, fulfilling social structures contract fewer infections, seek medical care less often and have stronger immune systems. It has been shown that cancer patients who join support groups experience better recovery from surgery and chemotherapy, live longer and are generally more positive about their disease outcome. We are social creatures; we need physical and emotional interaction to stay healthy. Infants raised in orphanages where little human touch and interaction was available failed to thrive, and illness and even mental retardation ensued. The slogan "Reach Out and Touch Someone" is a good one and we should do exactly that.

Smile Don't Frown

You may not even realize that you are frowning and that your shoulders are sloped as if they are bearing the weight of the world, but simply adjusting your posture and donning a smile will help you deal with the stressors around you. Try a simple test. Take two pieces of adhesive tape about two inches long and attach them to your forehead in a crisscross formation. Every time you frown, the tape will be tugged, providing you with a form of biofeedback. If deep frown lines are forming on your forehead, see them as an indicator of too much stress in your life. Relaxation techniques will work to diminish those wrinkles faster than miracle creams or cosmetic surgery.

NUTRIENTS PROTECT AGAINST THE EFFECTS OF STRESS

Adopt the super-immune diet recommended in chapter 5, include the nutritional supplements recommended in chapters 3 and 4 and add the following stress-effective remedies.

Moducare Sterinol

Whether stress is physical, emotional or social, it will cause the same physiological response in the body. Sterinol will increase DHEA levels naturally, increase the numbers and effectiveness of T-cells and natural killer cells to enhance immunity. At the same time, it will reduce the negative stress hormone cortisol and the pro-inflammatory agent interleukin-6, both known to inhibit good immune function.

Take 6 capsules each day for 1 week and 3 capsules each day thereafter on an empty stomach in the absence of dairy products to ensure maximum absorption.

Adrenal Extracts

Adrenal extracts are based on the concept that ingesting organ-specific extracts will help strengthen and promote repair of the targeted organ. Depending on the desired effect, extracts may be made from either the adrenal cortex or the whole adrenal gland.

Dosage for each product is different. Read the label and start off with half the recommended dose. If you are taking too much, you will feel agitated and may have trouble sleeping. Adjust accordingly. Use only high-quality adrenal extracts. We recommend Tyler and Klaire (see Appendix I).

Homeopathic Medicines

Homeopathy is an exceptionally safe form of natural medicine, which treats the whole individual, not just the symptoms from which the person is suffering. Homeopathy seeks to assist rather than oppose nature. It sees the disease state—the fever, inflammation, diarrhea, headache, etc.—as the body's attempt to return to a normal state. Based on the Laws of Similars, a homeopathic medicine—referred to as a remedy—is selected based on its ability to match the complete and unique symptom picture of the individual on all levels, including physical, mental and emotional symptoms. When administered, this similar homeopathic remedy mimics the prevailing symptoms the individual is already suffering. In so doing, it "duplicates" the sufferer's illness. This further alerts and kick-starts the body's sluggish defense system. Since no two similar states of discomfort can exist in the same body simultaneously, the body must throw one off, but because both disease states are so similar, the body does not differentiate between the two. The end result is the elimination of both states from the body and a return to health.

Homeopathic remedies are made from the plant, animal and mineral kingdoms. They are highly diluted, making them safe for all ages and for highly sensitive individuals. These medicines can be self-administered for simple, acute conditions. However, a qualified homeopathic practitioner should be consulted for more complex, chronic conditions.

Contact a homeopathic practitioner for a complete evaluation. Homeopathic remedies are excellent for treating emotionally based disorders. If you are suffering from a relationship breakup, repressed abuse or the death of a loved one, homeopathy can be an effective treatment. A caring homeopath can help get to the root of your stress-related health problems by taking a detailed case history. Homeopathy is person-specific, meaning that what works for one person may not work for another. We have seen excellent results with homeopathy.

Kava Extract

Anxiety is a state of abnormal or overwhelming apprehension marked by symptoms such as sweating, tension and increased heart rate. Some individuals experience panic attacks, a severe state of anxiety with symptoms so intense they cannot breathe, or they have chest pains so severe they think they are having a heart attack. Irritable bowel syndrome may also be exacerbated in times of stress and anxiety.

Kava kava is an excellent antianxiety herb. It is as effective as diazepam, commonly known as Valium, at reducing anxious states without the side effects frequently found with drug therapy.

A dose of 200 mg three times a day is recommended. Make sure that the product you purchase has 30 percent kavalactones (the active ingredient of kava kava).

EXERCISE AND IMMUNITY

Low to moderate exercise is beneficial to health and enhances immunity. Walking is the most potent immune-enhancing activity, providing movement to the body while clearing the mind. However, boost the intensity and duration of that same exercise and you will find that too much of a good thing can be bad. Overexercising causes stress on the immune system, resulting in higher-than-average colds, flu and poor recovery rates after exercise. Marathon runners are especially prone to negative side effects of strenuous, relentless exercise. Patrick Bouic and other researchers are discovering that the function of T-cells and natural killer cells is suppressed due to exercise overexertion. Suppression of the immune system results and this temporary susceptibility to microorganisms and viruses causes an increase in diseases including cancer.

Prominent immunologists and sports physiologists have been delving into the reasons why marathon runners are prone to colds and influenza during the period immediately following a marathon race. What they have found is that excessive physical stress causes tissue damage, and in response promotes an increase in the release of cortisol and pro-inflammatory factors, especially interleukin-6. Have you ever noticed that many marathon runners or those who take part in excessively demanding repetitive sports look aged? Without a good, solid diet and nutrient program, these people are actually speeding up the aging process—muscles start to waste and the skin wrinkles and sags. The body will find the nutrients it needs even if it has to steal them from muscles, bones and connective tissues. Make sure that you are getting the maximum nutrition for the amount of physical exercise output you are expending.

We are not saying don't exercise. We are saying that if you are going to take part in long-term, physically demanding exercise, take precautions and ensure that your immune system has the tools it needs to protect your body. We know that antioxidants are essential for athletes to curb any free radicals that are produced during a workout. Plant nutrients are also being recognized as important protectors in cases of intense activity. If you go to a gym or jog around the neighborhood on a poorly fed body you'll be damaging not only your muscles but also your immune system. Fitness starts with good wholesome food. You must provide the proper nutrients to protect your muscles and immunity.

Sport's nutrition science has become very sophisticated over the years. Solid nutrition is paramount to optimal physical performance. The super phytonutrient discussed below will ensure that you are able to recover from your workouts faster, allowing you to improve your performance over the long run. Post-workout colds, flu and aches and pains will also be alleviated. Please note that the focus here is on the immune system and preventing post-workout infections and improved recovery time, not muscle building. (If you are looking for information on muscle and fitness development, read Michael Colgan's *The Sports Nutrition Guide* and *The Power Program*, published by Apple Publishing, as well as Joyce L. Viedral's *Now or Never*, which focuses on women and fitness.)

STEROLS AND STEROLINS AND MARATHON RUNNERS

Marathon runners are a well-documented group of athletes who experience exercise-induced immune suppression. We know that the effect of exercise on the immune system depends on the duration and intensity of the exercise. High-intensity exercise for extended periods causes immune suppression, while low-intensity exercise is immune-enhancing. Many researchers have indicated an increase in white blood cell counts, while others have shown a reduction in the ability of those cells to function appropriately after high-intensity workouts. The type of immune suppression that occurs after a marathon race may be attributed to the lack of regulatory factors being released by helper T-cells, especially the powerful antiviral agent gamma-interferon. Also, increased levels of interleukin-6 are found in the blood and urine of athletes following strenuous workouts. Interleukin-6 is associated with high cortisol levels, low DHEA levels and reduced activity of natural killer cells. During this temporary immune-suppression period, microorganisms, especially viruses, have time to evade immune detection, and they become established, giving rise to infections.

Patrick Bouic and his research team have shown that plant sterols and sterolins are potent immune modulators (balance the immune system) capable of reversing abnormalities of the immune system. The aim of their study was to determine whether sterols and sterolins could inhibit the radical physiological changes seen in the blood of athletes and to ascertain whether these plant fats could decrease the inflammatory aspects, muscle pain and inflammation associated with the excessive exercise of marathon running.

A group of 20 athletes were recruited from a running club. The volunteers were recruited over a period of three weeks, two months prior to a 68-kilometer marathon event. The athletes were in good health and were selected on the basis of a questionnaire that took into consideration their previous running history and whether they were prone to upper respiratory tract or viral infections post-marathon. Four weeks prior to the event, all athletes gave blood, a careful history was recorded, including vitamin and mineral supplements, and use of antimicrobial agents during the preceding fourteen days. The volunteers were given either capsules containing sterols and sterolins (2 capsules to be taken three times a day) or a placebo. The study was double-blind and placebo-controlled with eight volunteers in the placebo group and nine in the active group. Three subjects were excluded because they did not return for the final blood workup. Routine tests included a full blood count and differential count and full liver function tests. Blood interleukin-6 levels were also evaluated.

Post-marathon results showed that the group treated with sterol and sterolin displayed a significant reduction in interleukin-6 compared to the placebo group. A profound effect was observed in the balance between cortisol and DHEA levels in the sterol and sterolin–treated group. Cortisol is an immune-suppressing hormone, and in the placebo group cortisol increased as expected; in the treated group it dropped. This cortisol decrease was accompanied by an increase in DHEA that was statistically significant. DHEA, the immune-regulating hormone is important in protecting the body from viral and bacterial infections, as well as inhibiting new tumors from forming. DHEA protects against lethal viral coxsackie B enterovirus or herpes type 2 and enterococcus faecalis infection. It has also been shown that cryptosporidium parvum infection was inhibited by DHEA treatment in rats. DHEA levels decline with age and it is proposed as one factor in immune dysregulation, such as raised interleukin-6 and the development of degenerative diseases including arthritis.

We know that a balance between the two types of helper T-cells is required for optimal immune health, and DHEA greatly enhances the action of T_H1 helper cells and the regulatory factors they release, including interleukin-2. In turn, DHEA increases the activity of cytotoxic T-cells and the number of helper T-cells called to battle, and decreases interleukin-4, which causes inflammation and tissue destruction. Sterols and sterolins are a precursor to pregnenolone and then to DHEA. This natural enhancement of DHEA is without the minor side effects of direct supplementation of DHEA, acne, hair growth and so on.

Due to the dysregulation of the immune system caused by an overdominance of T_H2 and underactivity of T_H1, it is found that DHEA levels are particularly low as a result. This is especially true in persons who use corticosteroid drugs for joint, cartilage or muscle injuries and autoimmune disorders such as lupus, rheumatoid arthritis and multiple sclerosis. Low DHEA levels are also seen in those with chronic fatigue syndrome and in individuals with poor recovery rates after intense workouts. DHEA is a super-immune hormone, and in order to stay young and healthy we must ensure adequate levels as we age.

The effects of intense exercise (a stressor) on the immune system has been under debate for many years. Most of the negative effects of overexercising can be attributed to excess cortisol production (the stress hormone), an imbalance in the ratio of T_H1 helper cells to T_H2 cells and a reduction in the antiaging super-immune hormone DHEA. Sterols and sterolins improve these parameters quickly, within several weeks. This non-toxic, affordable immune booster is the basis for immune health. If you add no other supplement to your diet, make sure you take Sterinol. Take 6 capsules a day for one week, and 3 capsules a day thereafter. This is a lifetime supplement that will protect you from opportunistic infections that are able to reproduce during times of stress.

———————

Fortified with the appropriate nutrients and supplements, allowed to recover sufficiently from physical, emotional and psychological stress, removed from the negative effects of environmental toxins, exercised and, yes, loved, your immune system is a powerful weapon against disease. Now that you've read and, we hope, assimilated, the tenets of the immune system cure, you have the power to heal yourself. Apply the recommendations in this book, and you will enjoy a life that is free from degenerative diseases; you will become increasingly responsive to your body's needs, and you will have committed yourself to a balanced lifestyle. Most important, you will have taken charge; *you* will be in control of your health.

Appendix I

PRODUCT MANUFACTURERS

Moducare® Sterinol™

WORLDWIDE DISTRIBUTORS:

Essential Sterolin Products (Pty) Ltd.
16th Road
Randjespark
Midrand, 1685
South Africa
Tel: 11-315-1430
Fax: 11-315-1462

IN CANADA:

Essential Phytosterolins Inc.
6 Commerce Crescent
Acton, Ontario L7J 2X3
Toll-Free: 877-297-7332
Tel: 519-853-1129
Fax: 519-853-4660
E-mail: info@moducare.com
Web site: www.moducare.com

Purity Professionals (professional distributor)
Division of Purity Life Health Products
2975 Lake City Way
Burnaby, British Columbia V5A 2Z6
Toll-free: 888-443-3323
Fax: 888-223-6111
E-mail: professional@puritylife.com

IN THE UNITED STATES:

Natural Balance, Inc. (health food store distributor)
P.O. Box 8002
3130 North Commerce Court
Castle Rock, Colorado 80104
Toll-free: 800-833-8737

Thorne Research (professional distributor)
P.O. Box 3200
Sandpoint, Idaho 83864
Tel: 208-263-1337
Toll-free: 800-228-1966
Fax: 208-265-2488
E-mail: info@thorne.com
Web site: www.thorne.com

Vitamins, Minerals, Amino Acids, Probiotics

IN CANADA:

Purity Professionals
Division of Purity Life Health Products
2975 Lake City Way
Burnaby, British Columbia V5A 2Z6
Toll-free: 888-443-3323
Fax: 888-223-6111
E-mail: professional@puritylife.com

IN THE UNITED STATES:

Klaire Laboratories, Inc.
1573 West Seminole
San Marcos, California 92069
Toll-free: 800-533-7255
Fax: 760-744-9364

––––––––––

Eskimo-3, Enzyme Supplements, Vitamins and Minerals

IN CANADA:

Tyler Encapsulations—Purity Professionals (Physicians) (see below)

Prevail Corporation—Purity Life Health Products
6 Commerce Crescent
Acton, Ontario L7J 2X3
Toll-free: 800-265-2615
Fax: 519-853-4660
Web site: www.puritylife.com

IN THE UNITED STATES:

Prevail Corporation (health food store distributor)
2204 North West Birdsdale
Gresham, Oregon 97030
Toll-free: 800-248-0885
Fax: 503-667-4790
E-mail: info@prevail.com
Web site: www.prevail.com

Tyler Encapsulations, Inc. (professional distributor)
2204 North West Birdsdale
Gresham, Oregon 97030
Toll-free: 800-869-9705
Fax: 503-666-4913
E-mail: info@tyler-inc.com
Web site: www.tyler-inc.com

Evening Primrose Oil, Efalex Focus, Omega Combination

IN CANADA:

Efamol Canada (1998) Ltd.
Scotia Centre
35 Webster Street
Kentville, Nova Scotia B4N 1H4
Toll-free: 800-539-3326
Fax: 902-678-2885
Web site: www.efamol.com

Flora Distributors Ltd. (health food store distributor)
7400 Fraser Park Drive
Burnaby, British Columbia V5J 5B9
Toll-free: 800-663-0617
Fax: 604-436-6060
E-mail: info@florahealth.com
Web Site: www.florahealth.com

Purity Professionals (professional distributor)
Division of Purity Life Health Products
2975 Lake City Way
Burnaby, British Columbia V5A 2Z6
Toll-free: 888-443-3323
Fax: 888-223-6111
E-mail: professional@puritylife.com

Gaia Herbal Preparations, Tinctures, Salves, etc.

IN CANADA:

Purity Life
6 Commerce Crescent
Acton, Ontario L7J 2X3
Tel: 519-853-3511
Toll-free: 800-265-2615
Fax: 519-853-4660
E-mail: info@puritylife.com

IN THE UNITED STATES:

Gaia Herbs
108 Island Ford Road
Brevard, North Carolina 28712
Toll-free: 800-831-7780
Fax: 800-717-1722

Udo's Choice Oil, Flax Oil, Beyond Greens, Udo's Wholesome Fast Food Blend

IN CANADA:

Flora Distributors Ltd.
7400 Fraser Park Drive
Burnaby, British Columbia V5J 5B9
Toll-free: 800-663-0617
Fax: 604-436-6060
E-mail: info@florahealth.com
Web Site: www.florahealth.com

IN THE UNITED STATES:

Flora Distributors Ltd.
P.O. Box 73
805 Badger Road East
Lynden, Washington 98264
Toll-free: 800-446-2110
Fax: 360-354-5355
E-mail: info@florahealth.com
Web Site: www.florahealth.com

Weleda Iscador (Mistletoe Preparation)

IN CANADA:

Purity Professionals
Division of Purity Life Health Products
2975 Lake City Way
Burnaby, British Columbia V5A 2Z6
Toll-free: 888-443-3323
Fax: 888-223-6111
E-mail: professional@puritylife.com

IN EUROPE:

Weleda AG
Heilmittel betriebe,
73503 Schwabisch Gmund
Germany
Tel: 49-717-191-9223
Fax: 49-717-191-9439

IN THE UNITED KINGDOM:

Weleda UK
Heanor Road
GB-Ilkeston/Derbyshire DE7 8DR
England
Tel: 44-115-944-8210

Omega Balance Oil, Flaxseed Oil, Pistachio Oil, Sunflower Oil, Garlic/Chili Flaxseed Oil, Pumpkin Seed Oil, Pumpkin Seed Spread

IN CANADA:

Omega Nutrition Canada Inc.
1924 Franklin Street
Vancouver, British Columbia V5L 1R2
Tel: 604-253-4677
Toll-free: 1-800-661-3529
Fax: 604-253-4893
E-mail: info@omegaflo.com
Web site: www.omegaflo.com

IN THE UNITED STATES:

Omega Nutrition U.S.A. Inc.
6515 Aldrich Road
Bellingham, Washington 98226
Tel: 360-384-1328
Toll-free: 1-800-661-3529
Fax: 360-384-0700
E-mail: info@omegaflo.com
Web Site: www.omegaflo.com

Sea-lutions Tuna Oil, Fish Oil, Salmon Oil, Shark Liver Oil

IN CANADA:

Ocean Nutrition Canada Ltd.
757 Bedford Highway
Bedford, Nova Scotia V4A 2Z7
Tel: 902-457-2399
Toll-free: 800-980-8889
Fax: 902-457-2357
Web site: www.ocean-nutrition.com

Green Drinks

IN CANADA:

Greens+ Canada
317 Adelaide Street West, Suite 501
Toronto, Ontario M5V 1P9
Tel: 416-977-3505
Toll-free: 877-500-7888
Fax: 416-977-4184
Web Site: www.greenspluscanada.com

IN THE UNITED STATES:

Green Foods Corporation
320 North Graves Avenue
Oxnard, California 93030
Tel: 805-983-7470
Toll-free: 800-777-4430
Web site: www.greenfoods.com

Healthy Directions, Inc.
7811 Montrose Road
Potomac, Maryland 28054-3394
Toll-free: 800-722-8008, ext. 2194

Orange Peel Enterprises, Inc.
2183 Ponce de Leon Circle
Vero Beach, Florida 32960
Toll-free: 800-643-1210
Web site: www.greensplus.com

Appendix II

RESOURCES

AIDS/HIV

AIDS Project Los Angeles (APLA)
1313 North Vine Street
Los Angeles, California 90028
Tel: 323-993-1600
Hotline: 800-367-2437
Fax: 323-993-1598
Web site: www.apla.org

AIDS Vancouver
Pacific AIDS Resource Centre
1107 Seymour Street
Vancouver, British Columbia V6B 5S8
Tel: 604-681-2122
TTY-TDD: 604-893-2215
Helpline: 604-687-2437
Fax: 604-893-2211

AmFAR (American Foundation for AIDS Research)
120 Wall Street, 13th Floor
New York, New York 10005
Tel: 212-806-1600
Fax: 212-806-1601
Web site: www.amfar.org

Canadian AIDS Society
130 Albert Street, Suite 900
Ottawa, Ontario H1P 5G4
Tel: 613-230-3580
Toll-free: 800-884-1058
Fax: 613-563-4998
Web site: www.cdnaids.ca

CDC National AIDS/HIV Hotline
Hotline (US only): 800-342-AIDS (342-2437)
Tel: 800-344-SIDA (Spanish)
E-mail: info@cdcnpin.org
Web sites: www.cdc.gov/nchstp/od/hotlines.htm
www.cdcnac.org/

Centers for Disease Control and Prevention
1600 Clifton Road, North East
Atlanta, Georgia 30333
Tel: 404-639-3311
E-mail: NCHSTP@cdc.gov
Web site: www.cdc.gov

National Association of People with AIDS
1413 K Street North West, 8th Floor
Washington, DC 20005
Tel: 202-898-0414
Hotline: 202-898-0414
Fax: 202-898-0435
E-mail: napwa@napwa.org
Web site: www.napwa.org

National Institute of Health (NIH)
P.O. Box 6421
Bethesda, Maryland 20892
Hotline: 800-874-2572
E-mail: NIHinfo@OD.NIH.gov
Web site: www.nih.gov

People with AIDS Coalition of New York
50 West 17th Street, 8th Floor
New York, New York 10011
Tel: 212-647-1415
Hotline: 212-647-1420
Fax: 212-647-1419
E-mail: newslineny@AOL.com

Stop AIDS Worldwide
2261 Old Middlefield Way
Mountain View, California 94043
Web site: www.stopaidsworldwide.org

Arthritis

American College of Rheumatology
1800 Century Place, Suite 250
Atlanta, Georgia 30345-4300
Tel: 404-633-3777
Fax: 404-633-1870
E-mail: acr@rheumatology.org
Web site: www.rheumatology.org

The Arthritis Society
National Office
393 University Avenue, Suite 1700
Toronto, Ontario M5G 1E6
Tel: 416-979-7228
Fax: 416-979-8366
E-mail: info@arthritis.ca
Web site: www.arthritis.ca

The Arthritis Trust of America
7111 Sweetgum Drive South West, Suite A
Fairview, Tennessee 37062-9384
Tel: 615-646-1030
E-mail: administration@arthritistrust.org
Web site: www.arthritistrust.org

Cancer

Canadian Cancer Society
10 Alcorn Avenue, Suite 200
Toronto, Ontario M4V 3B1
Tel: 416-961-7223
Fax: 416-961-4189

Cancer Victors Canada
6-625 Alpha Street
Victoria, British Columbia V8Z 1B5
Tel: 250-360-2988
Toll-free: 888-705-1777
Fax: 250-380-5125
E-mail: canvic@coastnet.com
Web site: www.cancervictors.com

———————

Diabetes

American Diabetes Association
National Office
1660 Duke Street
Alexandria, Virginia 22314
Toll-free: 800-342-2383
Fax: 703-549-6995
E-mail: customerservice@diabetes.org
Web site: www.diabetes.org

Canadian Diabetes Association
15 Toronto Street, Suite 800
Toronto, Ontario M5C 2E3
Tel: 416-363-3373
Toll-free: 800-BANTING
Fax: 416-363-3393
E-mail: info@cda-nat.org
Web site: www.diabetes.ca

Environmental Medicine, Allergy, and Clinical Immunology

AAEM (American Academy of Environmental Medicine)
10 East Randolph Street
New Hope, Pennsylvania 18938
Tel: 215-862-4544
Fax: 215-862-4583
E-mail: aaem@bellatlantic.net
Web site: www.aaem.com

Serammune Physicians Lab
14 Pidgeon Hill, Suite 300
Sterling, Virginia 20165
Toll-free: 800-553-5472
Fax: 703-450-2981
(ELISA/ACT allergy test)

Enzyme-Potentiated Desensitization (EPD)

American EPD Society
141 Paseo de Peralta
Santa Fe, New Mexico 87501
Tel: 505-983-8890
Fax: 505-820-7315
Web site: www.epdallergy.com

Fibromyalgia

British Columbia Fibromyalgia Society
Box 15455
Vancouver, British Columbia V6B 5B2
Tel: 604-540-0488

The Ontario Fibromyalgia Association
393 University Avenue, Suite 1700
Toronto, Ontario M5G 1E6
Tel: 416-979-7228
Fax: 416-979-8366
E-mail: info@arthritis.ca
Web site: www.arthritis.ca

Healing Spas

EcoMed Natural Health Spa
Pacific Shores Nature Resort, #515
1655 Stougler, R.R. #1, Box 50
Nanoose Bay, British Columbia V0R 2R0
Tel: 250-468-7133
Fax: 250-468-7135
E-mail: info@ecomedspa.com
Web site: www.ecomedspa.com

Mountain Trek Fitness Retreat & Health Spa
P.O. Box 1352
Ainsworth Hot Springs, British Columbia V0G 1A0
Tel: 250-229-5636
Fax: 250-229-5246
Toll-free: 800-661-5161
E-mail: wendy@hiking.com
Web site: www.hiking.com
 (Staffed by a resident naturopathic doctor and many health-care professionals. Offers a large array of up-to-date health-care alternatives.)

The Whitaker Wellness Institute
4321 Birch Street, Suite 100
Newport Beach, California 92660
Tel: 949-851-1550
Fax: 949-851-9970
(Staffed by Dr. Julian Whitaker and other physicians.)

Hepatitis

American Liver Foundation
75 Maiden Lane, Suite 603
New York, New York 10038-4810
Tel: 800-GO-LIVER (465-4837)
Tel: 888-4-HEP-ABC (443-7222)
Fax: 973-256-3214
E-mail: webmail@liverfoundation.org
Web site: www.liverfoundation.org

Hepatitis C Foundation of Canada
383 Huron Street
Toronto, Ontario M5S 2G5
Tel: 416-979-5855
Toll-free: 800-652-4372
Fax: 416-979-5856
E-mail: hecs@idirect.ca

Hepatitis Foundation International
30 Sunrise Terrace
Cedar Grove, New Jersey 07009
Tel: 800-891-0707
Fax: 973-857-5044
Web site: www.hefi.org

The Hepatitis C Foundation
1502 Russett Drive
Warminster, Pennsylvania 18974
Tel: 215-672-2606
Web site: www.hepcfoundation.org

The Hep C Connection
1741 Gaylord Street
Denver, Colorado 80206
Tel: 303-860-0800
Hep C Hotline: 800-522-HEPC
Hepatitis Help Line: 800-390-1202
E-mail: hepc-connection@worldnet.att.net
Web site: www.hepc-connection.org

Lupus

Lupus Foundation of America
1300 Piccard Drive, Suite 200
Rockville, Maryland 20850-4303
Tel: 301-670-9292
Toll-free: 800-558-0121
Fax: 301-670-9486
E-mail: lfanatl@aol.com
Web site: www.lupus.org

Naturopathic Medicine

American Association of Naturopathic Physicians
2366 Eastlake Avenue East, Suite 322
Seattle, Washington 98102
Tel: 206-323-7610
Web site: www.naturopathic.org

Canadian College of Naturopathic Medicine
2300 Yonge Street, 18th Floor
P.O. Box 2431
Toronto, Ontario M4P 1E4
Tel: 416-486-8584
Fax: 416-484-6821
E-mail: info@ccnm.edu
Web site: www.ccnm.edu

National College of Naturopathic Medicine
049 Southwest Porter Avenue
Portland, Oregon 97201
Tel: 503-499-4343
Fax: 503-499-0027
E-mail: admissions@ncnm.edu
Web site: www.ncnm.edu

Ontario Association of Naturopathic Doctors
4174 Dundas Street West, Suite 304
Etobicoke, Ontario
Tel: 416-233-2001
Fax: 416-233-2924

Physician Referrals

ACAM (American College for Advancement in Medicine)
23121 Verdugo Drive, Suite 204
Laguna Hills, California 92653
Toll-free (US only): 800-532-3688
E-mail: acam@acam.org
Web site: www.acam.org

Publications

Clinical Pearls
IT Services
Monthly issues
Tel: 916-483-1085
Fax: 916-483-1431
E-mail: office@clinicalpearls.com
Web site: www.clinicalpearls.com
Yearly subscription US$115

Colgan Chronicles
Colgan Institute
#204 – 523 Encinitas Boulevard
Encinitas, California 92024
Tel: 760-632-7722
Fax: 760-632-7375
Web site: www.colganchronicles.com
Eight issues a year
One-year subscription US$64
Canada, one-year subscription CDN$88
Canada, two-year subscription CDN$108

Life Extension Magazine
The Life Extension Foundation
995 South West 24th Street
Ft. Lauderdale, Florida 33315
Tel: 954-766-8433
Toll-free: 800-841-5433
Toll-free: 800-544-4440
E-mail: lef@lef.org
Web site: www.lef.org
One-year subscription US$75
Two-year subscription US$135

The Quarterly Review of Natural Medicine
Natural Product Research Consultants, Inc.
600 First Avenue, Suite 205
Seattle, Washington 98104
Tel: 973-762-0840
Web site: www.nprc.com

The Townsend Letter
911 Tyler Street
Port Townsend, Washington 98368-6541
Tel: 360-385-6021
Fax: 360-385-0699
E-mail: tldp@olympus.net
Web site: www.tldp.com
One-year subscription US$49
Two-year subscription US$88

Yoga

Himalayan Institute of Yoga, Science, and Philosophy
RR1 Box 400
Honesdale, Pennsylvania 18431
Tel: 717-253-5551
Toll-free: 800-822-4547

International Association of Yoga Therapists
109 Hillside Avenue
Mill Valley, California 94941
Tel: 415-381-0876

References

The books and articles listed below provide the details of the research on which we have based the recommendations contained in this book.

Chapter 2
Understanding Immunity

Becker, Wayne, and David Deamer. *The World of the Cell*, 2nd ed. (California: The Benjamin/Cummings Publishing Company Inc., 1991.)

Bland, Jeffrey. *Medical Applications of Clinical Nutrition*. (New Canaan, Connecticut: Keats Publishing, 1983.)

Peakman, Mark, and Diego Vergani. *Basic and Clinical Immunology*. (New York: Churchill Livingstone, 1997.)

Tortora, Gerard J., and Nicholas P. Anagnostakos. *Principles of Anatomy and Physiology*, 6th ed. (New York: Harper & Row, 1990.)

Chapter 3
Ten Nutritional Supplements to Boost Immunity

Bendich, A. 1989. "Carotenoids and the immune response." *Journal of Nutrition* 119: 112-15.

Bray, T.M., and Taylor, C.G. "Enhancement of tissue glutathione for antioxidant and immune functions in malnutrition." *Biochemical Pharmacology* 1994.

Buffington, C. K., G. G. Pourmotabbe and A. E. Kitabshi. 1993. "Case report: Amelioration of insulin resistance in diabetes with dehydroepiandrosterone." *American Journal of Medical Science* 306(5): 320-24.

Bum, M.K. et al. "Association of vitamin B_6 status with parameters of immune function in early HIV infection." *AIDS Journal*. 1991.

Buster, J. E. et al. 1992. "Postmenopausal steroid replacement with micronized dehydroepiandrosterone: preliminary oral bioavailability and dose proportionality studies." *American Journal of Obstetrics and Gynecology* 166(4): 1163-68.

Challem, J. "Zinc supplements can boost immunity, improve sense of taste some of the time." *The Nutrition Reporter* 1998: 9(10).

Eby, G. A. et al. 1984. "Reduction in duration of the common cold by zinc gluconate lozenges in a double-blind study." *Antimicrobial Agents Chemotherapy*.

Ewan, C. et al. 1979. "Ascorbic acid and cancer: A review." *Cancer Research*. 39: 663-81.

Folkers, K. et al. 1982. "Increase in levels of IgG in serum of patients treated with coenzyme Q_{10}." *Res Commun Chem Pathol Pharmacol*.

Fortes, C. 1995. "Aging, zinc and cell-mediated immune responses." *Aging Clinical and Experimental Research* 7:75-76.

Franceschi, S. et al. 1994. "Tomatoes and risk of digestive tract cancers." *International Journal of Cancer* 59: 181-84.

Garewal, H. S. et al. 1992. "A preliminary trial of beta-carotene in subjects infected with the human immunodeficiency virus." *Journal of Nutrition* 122: 728-32.

———. 1995. "Antioxidants in oral cancer prevention." *American Journal of Clinical Nutrition* 62 (supplement).

Giovanucci, E. et al. 1995. "Intake of carotenoids and retinol in relation to risk of prostate cancer." *Journal of the National Cancer Institute* 87: 1767-76.

Hemila, H. 1994. "Does vitamin C alleviate the symptoms of the common cold. A review of current evidence." *Scandinavian Journal of Infectious Diseases* 26: 4-5.

Heuser, G., and A. Vojdani. 1997. "Enhancement of natural killer cell activity and T and B cell function by buffered vitamin C in patients exposed to toxic chemicals: The role of protein Kinase C." *Immunopharmacology and Immunotoxicology.*

Hsu, J. M. 1981. "Lead toxicity as related to glutathione metabolism." *Journal of Nutrition* 3: 26-33.

Jeng, Kee-Ching G. et al. 1996. "Supplementation with vitamin C and E enhances cytokine production by peripheral blood mononuclear cells in healthy adults." *American Journal of Clinical Nutrition.*

Jolly, P. et al. 1996. "Vitamin A deficiency in HIV infection and AIDS." *AIDS Journal.*

Julius, M. et al. 1994. "Glutathione and morbidity in a community-based sample of elderly." *Journal of Clinical Epidemiology.*

Kiremidijian-Schumacher, L. et al. 1994. "Supplementation with selenium and human immune cell function. Its effect on cytotoxic lymphocytes and natural killer cells." *Biological Trace Element Research* 41: 115-27.

Knekt, P. et al. 1988. "Serum vitamin E level and risk of female cancers." *International Journal of Epidemiology* 17: 281-86.

Leblhuber, F. et al. 1993. "Age and sex differences of dehydroepiandrosterone sulfate (DHEAS) and cortisol plasma levels in normal controls and Alzheimer's disease." *Psychopharmacology* 111(1): 23-26.

Levander, O., and M. Beck. 1996. "Selenium deficiency results in viral virulence." *Journal of the American College of Nutrition.*

Lockwood, K. et al. 1994. "Partial and complete regression of breast cancer in patients in relation to dosage of coenzyme Q_{10}." *Biochemical and Biophysical Research Communications* 199: 1504-8.

Mara, J. et al. 1994. "Glutathione and morbidity in a community-based sample of elderly." *Journal of Clinical Epidemiology* 47: 1021-36.

Messina, M. and S. Barnes. 1991. "The role of soy products in reducing risk of cancer." *Journal of the National Cancer Institute* 83: 541-42.

Murata, T. et al. 1994. "Effect of long-term administration of beta-carotene on lymphocyte subsets in humans." *American Journal of Clinical Nutrition* 60: 587-602.

Prasad, A. S. 1980. "Effect of vitamin E supplementation on leukocyte function." *American Journal of Clinical Nutrition* 33: 606.

———. 1995. "Zinc: an overview." *Nutrition Reviews.*

Regelson, W. and M. Kalimi. 1994. "Dehydroepiandrosterone (DHEA)—the multifunctional steroid." *Annals of the New York Academy of Science* 719: 564-75.

Sandstead, Harold, and Nancy Alcock. 1997. "Zinc: An essential and unheralded nutrient." *Journal of Laboratory and Clinical Medicine.*

Sazawal, S. et al. 1998. "Zinc supplementation reduces the incidence of acute lower respiratory infections in infants and preschool children: A double-blind, controlled study." *Pediatrics* 102: 1-5.

Tarp, U. et al. 1985. "Selenium treatment in rheumatoid arthritis." *Scandinavian Journal of Rheumatology.*

Van Vollenhoven, R. F., E. G. Engelman, and J. L. McGuire. 1994. "An open study of DHEA in SLE." *Arthritis and Rheumatology* 37(9): 1305-10.

Wald, N. J. et al. 1984. *British Journal of Cancer.*

Yu, S. Y. et al. 1985. "Regional variation of cancer mortality incidence and its relation to selenium levels in China." *Biological Trace Element Research* 7: 21-29.

Chapter 4
Phytonutrients: Powerful Immune System Protection

Albertazzi, P. et al. 1998. "The effect of dietary soy supplementation on hot flashes." *Obstet Gynecol* 91(1): 6-11.

Bjorkhem, I. and K. M. Boberg. "Inborn errors in bile and biosynthesis and storage of sterols other than cholesterol." In *The Metabolic and Molecular Bases of Inherited Disease*, edited by C. R. Scriver, A. L. Beaudet, W. S. Sly and D. Valle, vol 2. 7th ed., pp. 2073-99. London: McGraw-Hill (1995).

Garewal, H. S. et al. 1992. "A preliminary trial of beta-carotene in subjects infected with the human immunodeficiency virus." *Journal of Nutrition* 122: 728-32.

Gartner, C. et al. 1997. "Lycopene is more bioavailable from tomatoe paste than from fresh tomatoes." *American Journal of Clinical Nutrition* 66(1): 116-22.

Giovannucci, E., et al. 1995. "Intake of carotenoids and retinol in relation to risk of prostate cancer." *Journal of the National Cancer Institute* 87(23): 1767-76.

Jang, M. et al. 1997. "Cancer chemopreventive activity of resveratrol, a natural product derived from grapes." *Science* 275: 218-20.

Ling W. H. and P. J. H. Jones. 1995. "Dietary phytosterols: a review of metabolism, benefits and side effects." *Life Sci.* 57: 195-206.

Michnovicz, J. et al. 1997. "Changes in levels of urinary estrogen metabolites after oral indole-3-carbinol treatment in humans." *Journal of the National Cancer Institute* 89(10): 718-23.

Nishida, Y., H. Sumi and H. Mihara. 1984. *Cancer Research.* 44: 3324-29.

Oritz de Montellano, P. R. 1984. *Ann. Rep. Med. Chem.* 19: 201-11.

Potischman, N. et al. 1990. "Breast cancer and dietary and plasma concentrations of carotenoids and vitamin A." *American Journal of Clinical Nutrition* 52: 909-15.

Sakiyama H. et al. 1984. *Cancer Research.* 44: 2023-32.

Valhouny, G. V., and D. Kritchevsky. 1981. "Plant and Marine Sterols and Cholesterol, *Nutrition Pharmacology* 95: 32-69.

Weihrauch, J. L., and J. M. Gardener. 1978. "Sterol content of foods of plant origin." *J. Am. Dietetic Assoc.* 73:39-47, and cited references.

Chapter 5
Disease Prevention: How to Optimize Immunity with Nutrition

Aviram, M. and K. Eigs. 1995. "Dietary olive oil reduces low-density lipoprotein uptake by macrophages and decreases the susceptibility of the lipoprotein to undergo lipid peroxidation." *Annals of Nutrition and Metabolism* 37: 75-89.

Barone, J. et al. 1989. "Dietary fat and natural killer cell activity." *American Journal of Clinical Nutrition.* 50: 861-67.

Bianchi-Salvadori, B. and R. Vesely. 1995. "Lactic acid bacteria and intestinal microflora." *Microecology and Therapy* 25: 247-55.

Block, G. 1991. "Vitamin C and cancer prevention: The epidemiologic evidence." *American Journal of Clinical Nutrition* 53: 270-282.

Calomme, M. et al. 1995. "Seleno-lactobacillus: an organic selenium source." *Biological Trace Element Research* 47: 379-83.

Carper, J. *Food, Your Miracle Medicine.* (New York: Harper Perennial, 1993.)

Caygill, C. P. et al. 1996. "Fat, fish, fish oil and cancer. *British Journal of Cancer* 74: 159-164.

Challem J. 1998. "The paleolithic diet versus modern diet: you are what your ancestors ate." *The Nutrition Reporter* 9: 1.

——. 1998. "Soy isoflavones for women's health." *Nutrition Science News* 3(9).

DeStefani, E. et al. 1997. "Dietary fiber and risk of breast cancer." *Nutrition and Cancer* 28: 14-19.

Eaton, S. B., S. B. Eaton III, and M. J. Konner. 1997. "Paleolithic nutrition revisited: A twelve-year retrospective on its nature and implications." *European Journal of Clinical Nutrition* 51: 207-16.

Erasmus, U. *Fats That Heal, Fats That Kill.* (Burnaby, British Columbia: Alive Books, 1997.)

Ernst, E. 1997. "Can allium vegetables prevent cancer?" *Phytomedicine* 4: 79-83.

Francheschi, S. et al. 1996. "Intake of macronutrients and risk of breast cancer." *The Lancet* 347: 1351.

——. 1994. "Tomatoes and risk of digestive tract cancers." *International Journal of Cancer* 59: 181-84.

Garewal, H. 1995. "Antioxidants in oral cancer prevention." *American Journal of Clinical Nutrition.*

Gerhauser, C. et al. 1997. "Cancer chemoprevention potential of sulforamate, a novel analogue of sulforaphane that induces phase 2 drug metabolizing enzymes." *Cancer Research* 57: 272-78.

Getchell, K. 1991. "The role of soy products in reducing risk of cancer." *Journal of the National Cancer Institute* 83: 8.

Gould, G. G. 1955. "Absorbability of beta-sitosterol." *The New York Academy of Sciences* 18: 129-34.

Haddad, J. G. et al. 1970. "Circulating phytosterols in normal females, lactating mothers and breast cancer patients." *Clinical Endocrinology* 30: 174-80.

Hannigan, B. 1994. "Diet and immune function." *British Journal of Biomedical Sciences* 51: 252-59.

Howe, G. R. et al. 1990. "Dietary factors and risk of breast cancer." Combined Analysis of 12 Case Control Studies. *Journal of the National Cancer Institute* 82: 561-69.

Jankun, J. et al. 1997. "Why drinking green tea could prevent cancer." *Nature* 387: 501.

Kinsella, J. and B. Lokesh. 1990. "Dietary lipids, eicosanoids, and the immune system." *Critical Care Medicine* 18: 1

La Vecchia, C. et al. 1996. "Olive oil and breast cancer risk in Italy." *Nutrition Research Newsletter* 15: 12.

Li, G. et al. 1995. "Anti-proliferative effects of garlic constituents in cultured human breast cancer cells." *Oncology Reports* 2: 787-91.

Mark, M. and S. Barnes. 1991. "The role of soy products in reducing risk of cancer." 83: 541-46.

Martin-Moreno, J. M. et al. 1994. "Dietary fat, olive oil intake and breast cancer risk." *International Journal of Cancer* 58: 774-80.

Nair, P. P. et al. 1984. "Diet, nutrition intake and metabolism in populations at high and low risk for colon cancer." *The American Journal of Clinical Nutrition* 40: 927-30.

Newberne, P. M. 1981. "Dietary fat, immunological response and cancer in rats." *Cancer Research* 41: 3783-85.

Pauling, L. *How to Live Longer and Feel Better.* (New York: W.H. Freeman & Company, 1986.)

Quillan, P. and N. Quillan. 1994. *Beating Cancer with Nutrition.* (Tulsa, Oklahoma: Nutrition Times Press, 1994.)

Ringsdorf, W. R., Jr. et al. 1976. "Sucrose, neutrophilic phagocytosis and resistance to disease." *Dental Survey* 52: 46-48.

Salminen, E. et al. *Adverse Effects of Pelvic Radiation.* Fifth International Meeting on Progress in Radio-oncology. May 1995. 10-14:501-4.

Schuler, I. et al. 1990. "Soybean phosphatidylcholine vesicles containing plant sterols: A fluorescence anisotropy study." *Biochimica et Biophysica Acta* 1028: 82-88.

Shahani and Fernandes. 1990. "Anticarcinogenic and immunological properties of dietary lactobacilli." *Journal of Food Protection* 53: 704-10.

Shahani et al. 1993. "Benefits of yogurt." *International Journal of Immunotherapy* 9(1): 65-68.

Stimpel, M. et al. 1984. "Macrophage activation and induction of macrophage cytotoxicity by purified polysaccharide fraction from the plant echinaceae purpurea." *Infection and Immunity* 46: 845-49.

Teas, J. 1981. "The consumption of seaweed as a protective factor in the etiology of breast cancer." *Medical Hypotheses* 7: 601-13.

Thresiamma, K. et al. 1996. "Protective effect of curcumin, ellagic acid and bixin on radiation-induced toxicity." *Indian Journal of Experimental Biology* 34: 845-47.

Verhoeven, D.T. et al. 1996. "Epidemiological studies on brassica vegetables and cancer risk." *Cancer Epidemiological Biomarkers* 5: 743-48.

Wang, C. et al. 1994. "Lignans and flavonoids inhibit aromatase enzyme in human preadipocytes." *Journal of Steroid Biochemistry and Molecular Biology* 50: 205-12.

Weihrauch, J. L. and J. M. Gardner. 1978. "Sterol content of foods of plant origin." *Journal of The American Dietetic Association* 73: 39-47.

Wong, J. L. 1986. "Cancer and chemicals and vegetables." *Chemtech* 16: 100-7.

Yip, I. et al. 1996. "Nutritional approaches to the prevention of prostate cancer progression." *Advances in Experimental Medicine and Biology* 399: 173-81.

Yu, T. G. et al. 1994. "Reduced risk of esophageal cancer associated with green tea consumption." *Journal of the National Cancer Institute* 86: 855-58.

Yudkin, J. *Sweet and Dangerous*. (Peter H. Wyden Publishers, 1972.)

Zava, D. T. and G. Euwe. 1997. "Estrogenic and antiproliferative properties of genistein and other flavonoids in human breast cancer cells in vitro." *Nutrition and Cancer* 27: 31-40.

Zheng, W. et al. 1996. "Tea consumption and cancer incidence in a prospective cohort study of postmenopausal women." *American Journal of Epidemiology* 144: 175-82.

——. 1995. "Retinol, antioxidant vitamins, and cancers of the upper digestive tract in a prospective cohort study of postmenopausal women." *American Journal of Epidemiology* 142: 955-60.

——. 1995. "Over 50 million drink water failing health standards." *Nutrition Week*.

Chapter 6
The Mind and the Immune System

Ader, R. et al. 1995. "Psychneuoimmunology: interactions between the nervous system and the immune system." *Lancet* 14: 988-93.

Bartrop, R.W. et al. 1977. "Depressed lymphocyte function after bereavement." *Lancet* 8016: 834-36.

Beasley, J. D. and J. Swift. 1989. Kellogg Report–the Impact of Nutrition, Environment and Lifesyle on the Health of Americans.

Blalock, E. J. 1984. "The immune system as a sensory organ." *Journal of Immunology* 132: 1067-70.

Chrousos, G. P., and P. W. Gold. 1992. "The concepts of stress and stress system disorder." *The Journal of the American Medical Association* 267(9): 1249.

Cohen, S. and B. S. Rabin. 1998. "Psychological stress, immunity and cancer." *Journal of the National Cancer Institute* 90: 3-4.

Cohen, S., D. A. Tyrrel, and A. P. Smith. 1991. "Psychological stress and susceptibility to the common cold." *New England Journal of Medicine* 325: 606-12.

Jahnke, R. 1991. "The most profound medicine—Part II and Part III: Physiological mechanisms operating in the human system during the practice of qigong and yoga pranayama." *Townsend Letter for Doctors* 91-92; 124-30; 281-85.

Kiecolt-Glaser, J. K. et al. 1986. "Modulation of cellular immunity in medical students." *Journal of Behavorial Medicine* 9(1): 19.

Moyers, B. *Healing and The Mind.* (New York: Doubleday, 1993.)

Rasmussen, A. F., Jr. 1969. "Emotions and immunity." *Annals of the New York Academy of Sciences* 164(2): 458-62.

Schleifer, S. J. et al. 1983. "Suppression of lymphocyte stimulation following bereavement." *The Journal of the American Medical Association* 250(3): 374-77.

Siegel, B. S. *Peace, Love and Healing.* (New York: Harper and Row, 1989.)

Soloman, G. F. 1969. "Emotions, stress, the central nervous system and immunity." *Annals of the New York Academy of Sciences* 164(2): 335-43.

Stone, A. A. et al. 1987. "Evidence that secretory IgA antibody is associated with daily mood." *Journal of Personality and Social Psychology* 52(5): 988-93.

Chapter 7
Cancer and Immunity

Allison, A. C., J. C. Lee, E. M. Eugui. 1995. "Pharmacological regulation of the production of the pro inflammatory cytokines TNF-a and IL-1ß." In *Human Cytokines: Their Role in Disease and Therapy*, edited by B. Aggarwal and R. Puri. *Blackwell Science* 689-713.

Beisel, W. R. 1991. "Single nutrients and immunity." *American Journal of Clinical Nutrition* 53: 386.

Breen, E. C. et al. 1990. "Infection with HIV is associated with elevated IL6 levels and production." *Journal of Immunology* 144: 480-84.

Burkitt, D. P. et al. 1972."Effect of dietary fibre on stools and transit times and its role in the causation of disease." *Lancet* 2: 1408-11.

Caygill, C. P. et al. 1996. "Fat, fish oil and cancer." *British Journal of Cancer* 74: 159-64.

Chiara, G. et al. 1969. "Inhibition of mouse sarcoma 180 by polysaccharides from Lentinus edodes." *Nature* 222: 637-38.

Cohen, B. I. et al. 1974. "The effect of dietary bile acids, cholesterol and B sitosterol upon formation of coprostanol and 7-dehydroxylation of bile acids in the rat." *Lipids* 9: 1027-29.

Day, E. A. et al. 1969. "Tumor sterols." *Metabolisms* 18: 646-51.

Gerhauser, C. et al. 1997. "Cancer chemoprevention potential of sulforamate, a novel analogue of sulforaphane that induces phase 2 drug-metabolizing enzymes." *Cancer Research* 57: 272-78.

Gould, R. G. et al. 1969. "Absorbability of B-sitosterol in humans." *Metabolism* 18: 652-62.

Haddad, J. G. et al. 1970. "Circulation phytosterols in normal females, lactating mothers and breast cancer patients." *Clinical Endocrinology* 30: 174-80.

Hartwell, J. L. "Types of anticancer agents isolated from plants." *Cancer Treatment* 60: 1031-67.

Hathcock, J. N. et al. 1990. "Micronutrients and immune function." *Annals of the New York Academy of Science* 587: 257-58.

Kalimi, M. et al. 1994. "Anti-glucocorticoid effects of dehydroepiandrosterone (DHEA)." *Molecular and Cellular Biochemistry* 131: 99-104.

Katiyar, S. et al. 1997. "Protective effects of silymarin against photocarcinogenesis in a mouse model." *Journal of the National Cancer Institute* 89: 556-65.

Linker-Israeli, M. et al. 1991. "Elevated levels of endogenous IL6 in systemic lupus erythematosus." *Journal of Immunology* 147: 117-23.

Meilles, M. J. et al. 1977. "Phytosterols and cholesterol in malignant and benign breast tumors." *Cancer Research* 27: 3034.

Meittinen, T. A., and S. Tarpila. 1978. "Fecal B-sitosterol in patients with diverticular disease of the colon in vegetarians." *Scandinavian Journal of Gastroenterology* 13: 573-76.

Nair, P. P. et al. 1984. "Diet, nutrition intake and metabolism in populations at high and low risk for colon cancer." *The American Journal of Clinical Nutrition*. 40: 927-30.

Namba, H. 1996. "Maitake D-fraction, healing and preventing potential for cancer." *Townsend Letter for Doctors and Patients*. 84-85.

Namba, H. et al. 1995. "Activity of maitake D-fraction to inhibit carcinogenesis and metastasis." *Annals of the New York Academy of Sciences* 768: 243-45.

O'Garra, A. 1989. "Interleukins and the immune system one." *Lancet* [April] 29:943-47.

———. 1989. "Interleukins and the immune system two." *Lancet* [May] 6: 1003-5.

Phillips, R. L. 1975. "Role of life-style and dietary habits in risk of cancer among Seventh-Day Adventists." *Cancer Research* 35-3513-22.

Raicht, R. F. et al. 1980. "Protective effect of plant sterols against chemically induced colon tumors in rats." *Cancer Research* 40: 403-5.

Reuben, J., and M. Larocco. 1988. "Cellular immune responses in acquired immunodeficiency syndrome." *Clinical Lab Sci*. 1: 90-95.

Roitt, I. *Essential Immunology*, 7th ed. (Blackwell Scientific Publication, 1991.)

Schwartz, A. G. and L. L. Pashko. 1993. "Cancer chemoprevention with the adrenocortical steroid dehydroepiandrosterone and structural analogs." *Journal of Cellular Biochemistry* 17: 73-79.

Simone, C. B. *Cancer and Nutrition*. (Garden City, New York: Avery, 1992.)

Verhoeven, D. T. et al. 1996. "Epidemiological studies on brassica vegetables and cancer risk." *Cancer Epidemiological, Biomarkers and Prevention* 5: 733-47.

Watson, J., and D. Mochizuki. 1980. "Interleukin 2: A class of T cell growth factors." *Immunology Review* 51: 257-78.

Yamada, H. et al. 1987. "Effects of phytosterols on anticomplementary activity." *Chemical Pharmacy Bulletin* 35(12)4851-55.

Yun, T. K., and S. Y. Choi. 1995. "Preventive effect of ginseng intake against various human cancers: A case control study on 1,987 pairs." *Cancer Epidemiology, Biomarkers and Prevention* 4: 401-8.

Yun, T. K. et al. 1993. "Cohort study on ginseng intake and cancer for population over 40 years old in ginseng production areas." Meeting Abstract. Second International Cancer Chemo Prevention Conference. Berlin, Germany.

Chapter 8
Protect Your Prostate

Berges, R. R., J. Windeler et al. 1995. "Randomized, placebo-controlled, double-blind clinical trial of (B-sitosterol in patients with benign prostatic hyperplasia." *Lancet* 345: 1529-32.

Berry, S. J. et al. 1994. "The development of human benign prostatic hyperplasia with age." *Journal of Urology* 132: 474-79.

Buck, A. C. 1996. "Phytotherapy for the prostate." *British Journal of Urology* 78: 325-36.

Finasteride Study Group. 1993. "Finasteride (MK-906) in the treatment of benign prostatic hyperplasia." *Prostate* 22: 291-99.

Fleming, C. et al. 1993. "A decision analysis of alternative treatment strategies for clinically localized prostate cancer." *Journal of the American Medical Association* 269 (2): 2650-58.

Klippel, K. F. 1997. "A multicentric, placebo-controlled double-blind clinical trial of B-sitosterol (phytosterol) for the treatment of benign prostatic hyperplasia." 80: 427-32.

McDougal, Scott. *Prostate Disease*. (New York: Times Books, 1996.)

Morton, M. S. et al. "The preventive role of diet in prostatic disease." *British Journal of Urology* 77: 491-93.

Murray, M. T., and J. E. Pizzorno. *Encyclopedia of Natural Medicine*. (California: Prima Publishing, 1991.)

Quillan, P. and N. Quillan. *Beating Cancer with Nutrition*. (Tulsa, Oklahoma: Nutrition Times Press, 1994.)

Reichert, R. 1995. "B-sitosterols in the management of BPH." *Quarterly Review of Natural Medicine*. 179-180.

Schachter, M. 1996. "Alternative Approaches to Prostate Cancer." *Integrative Medicine Healthworld Online*.

Schmidt, R. *Traditional Foods Are Your Best Medicines*. (Stratford, Conn.: Ocean View Publications, 1987.)

Walker, M. 1991. "Serenoa repens (saw palmetto) extract relief for benign prostatic hypertrophy." *Townsend Letter for Doctors*. [Feb/March]

Yip, I. et al. 1996. "Nutritional approaches to the prevention of prostate cancer progression." *Advances in Experimental Medicine and Biology* 399: 173-81.

Chapter 9
Autoimmune Diseases

Adam, O. 1995. "Antiinflammatory diet in rheumatic diseases." *European Journal of Clinical Nutrition* 49: 703-17.

Behr, S. M., and S. A. Porcelli. 1995. "Mechanisms of autoimmune disease induction." *Arthritis and Rheumatism* 38(4): 458-76.

Bigazzi, P. E. 1997. "Autoimmunity caused by xenobiotics." *Toxicology* 119: 1-21.

Bland, Jeffrey S. Health Comm International Seminar. 1998.

Bouic, P. J. D. "Sterols/sterolins, the natural, non-toxic immunomodulators and their role in the control of rheumatoid arthritis." Preliminary research results paper, 1998.

Bradley, J. D. et al. 1991. "Comparison of an antiinflammatory dose of ibuprofen, an analgesic dose of ibuprofen, and acetaminophen in the treatment of patients with osteoarthritis of the knee." *The New England Journal of Medicine* 325: 87-91.

D'Adamo, Peter J. *4 Blood Types, 4 Diets, Eat Right For Your Type.* (New York: G.P. Putnam's Sons, 1996.)

D'Ambrosio, E. et al. 1981. "Glucosamine sulfate: A controlled clinical investigation in arthrosis." *Pharmatherapeutica* 2(8): 504–10.

Dexter P., and K. Brandt. 1994. "Distribution and predictors of depressive symptoms of osteoarthritis." *The Journal of Rheumatology* 21(2): 279-86.

Dixon, J. et al. "Second-line agents in the treatment of rheumatic diseases." (New York: Marcel Dekker, 1992.)

Fabender, H. M. et al. 1994. "Glucosamine sulfate compared to ibuprofen in osteoarthritis of the knee." *Osteoarthritis and Cartilage* 2(1): 61-69.

Gay, G. 1990. Another side effect of NSAIDs. *Journal of the American Medical Association* 264(20): 2677-78.

Gecht, M. R. et al. 1996. "A survey of exercise beliefs and exercise habits among people with arthritis." *Arthritis Care and Research* 9(2): 82-88.

Gupta, M. B. et al. 1980. "Anti-inflammatory and antipyretic activities of B-sitosterol." *Planta Medica* 339: 157-63.

Hodgkinson, R., and D. Woolf. 1979. "A five year clinical trial of indomethacin in osteoarthritis of the hip joint." *ACTA Orthop Scand.* 50: 169-70.

Host, A. 1997. "Cow's milk allergy." *Journal of the Royal Society of Medicine* 90: 34-39 [supplement].

Jefferies, W. M. 1991. "Cortisol and immunity." *Medical Hypotheses* 34: 203.

Kitts, D. et al. 1997. "Adverse reactions to food constituents: Allergy intolerance and autoimmunity." *Canadian Journal of Physiology and Pharmacology* 75: 241-54.

McNeal, R. L. 1990. "Aquatic therapy for patients with rheumatic disease." *Rheumatic Disease Clinics of North America* 16(4): 915-43.

Moreland, L. W. 1997. "Treatment of rheumatoid arthritis with recominant human tumor necrosis factor receptor (p75) Fc fusion." *New England Journal of Medicine* 337(3): 141-47.

Murray, M. T. *Arthritis: How You Can Benefit from Diet, Vitamins, Minerals, Herbs, Exercise and Other Natural Methods.* (California: Prima Publishing, 1994.)

———. *Encyclopedia of Nutritional Supplements.* (Rocklin, California: Prima Publishing, 1998.)

Murray, Michael, and Joseph Pizzorno. *Encyclopedia of Natural Medicine*, 2nd ed. (Rocklin, California: Prima Publishing, 1998.)

Newman, N. M. et al. 1985. "Acetabular bone destruction related to nonsteroidal antiinflammatory drugs." *Lancet* 2: 11-14.

Nossal, G. J. V. 1989. "Immunological tolerance: Collaboration between antigen and lymphokines." *Science* 245: 147-53.

Perneger, T. V. et al. 1994. "Risk of kidney failure associated with the use of acetaminophen, aspirin, and nonsteroidal anitiinflammatory drugs." *New England Journal of Medicine* 331(25): 1675-79.

Pipitone, V. R. 1991. "Chondroprotection with chondroitin sulfate." *Drugs in Experimental and Clinical Research* 17(1): 3-7.

Rennie, J. 1990. "The body against itself." *Scientific America* [December] 76-85.

Samuel, M. P. et al. 1995. "Fast food arthritis, a clinic pathologic study of post-salmonella reactive arthritis." *Journal of Rheumatology* 22: 1947-52.

Theodosakis, J. *The Arthritis Cure, New Hope For Beating Arthritis.* (New York: St. Martin's Press, 1997.)

Traut, E. F. and C. B. Thrift. 1969. "Obesity in arthritis: Related factors, dietary factors." *Journal of the American Geriatric Society* 17: 710-17.

Van Vollenhoven, R. F. et al. 1994. "An open study of dehydroepiandrosterone in systemic lupus erythematosus." *Arthritis and Rheumatism* 37: 1305-10.

Vaz, A. L. 1982. "Double-blind clinical evaluation of the relative efficacy of ibuprofen and glucosamine sulphate in the management of osteoarthrosis of the knee in out-patients." *Current Medical Research and Opinion* 8(3): 145-49.

Yamamoto, M. et al. 1991. "Anti-inflammatory active constituents of Aloe arborescens Miller." *Agric. Biol. Chem.* 55(6): 1627-29.

Chapter 10
Allergies and the Immune System

Baumgardner, D. J. 1991. "Persistent urticaria caused by a common coloring agent." *Postgrad med.* 85(6): 265.

Bittiner, S. B. et al. 1988. "A double-blind, randomised, placebo-controlled trial of fish oil in psoriasis." *Lancet* 1(8582): 378-80.

Burton Goldberg Group. *Alternative Medicine: The Definitive Guide.* (Puyallup, Washington: Future Medicine Publishing, 1994.)

Chandra, R. K. 1983. "Nutrition, immunity, and infection: Present knowledge and future directions." *Lancet* 1(8326): 688.

Cogan, D. G. et al. 1984. "Aldose reductase and complications of diabetes." *Annals of Internal Medicine* 40: 184-85.

Collip, P. J. et al. 1975. "Pyridoxine treatment of childhood bronchial asthma." *Annuals of Allergy* 35: 93-97.

Delport, R. et al. 1988. "Vitamin B_6 nutritional status in asthma: The effect of theophylline therapy on plasma pyridoxal-5-phosphate and pyridoxal levels." *International Journal of Vitamin Research* 58(1): 67-72.

Galland, L. 1986. "Increased requirements for essential fatty acids in atopic individuals, a review with clinical descriptions." *American Journal of Clinical Nutrition* 5: 213-28.

Hertog, M. L., and P. H. Hollman. 1996. "Potential health effects of the dietary flavonol quercetin." *European Journal of Clinical Nutrition* 50: 63-71.

Hodge, L. et al. 1996. "Consumption of oily fish and childhood asthma risk." *Medical Journal of Austria* 163(3): 137-40.

Hoj, L. et al. 1981. "A double-blind controlled trial of elemental diet in severe, perennial asthma." *Allergy* 36:257-62.

———. 1989. "Inflammation and nutrition." *Medical Nutrition* (Fall): 42-45.

Kamimierczak, W., and B. Diamant. 1978. "Mechanisms of histamine release in anaphylactic and anaphylactoid reactions." *Prog Allergy* 24: 295.

Lee, T. H., and J. P. Arm. 1989. "Modulation of the allergic response by fish oil lipids and eicosatrienoic acid." *Prog Clin Biol Res.* 297: 57-69.

Lichtenstein, L. M. 1993. "Allergy and the immune system." *Scientific America* (Sept): 116-24.

Peakman, M., and D. Vergani. *Basic and Clinical Immunology.* (New York: Churchill Livingstone, 1997.)

Rosenbaum, M. and M. Susser. *Solving the Puzzle of Chronic Fatigue Syndrome.* (Tacoma, Washington: Life Sciences Press, 1992.)

Schwartz, J. 1994. "The relationship of dietary fish intake to level of pulmonary function in the first National Health and Nutrition Survey." *European Respiratory Journal* 7(10): 1821-24.

Tixier, J. M. et al. 1984. "Evidence by in vivo and in vitro studies that binding of pycnogenols to elastin affects its rate of degradation by elastases." *Biochemical Pharmacology* 33(24): 3933-39.

Varma, S. D. et al. 1977. "Diabetic cataracts and flavonoids." *Science* 195: 205.

Venge, P. et al. 1987. "Eosinophil activation in allergic disease." *Archives of Allergy and Applied Immunology* 82: 333.

Voelker, R. 1995. "Ames agrees with mom's advice: Eat your fruits and vegetables." *The Journal of the American Medical Association* 273(14): 1077-78.

Werbach, M. *Healing Through Nutrition.* (New York: Harper Collins, 1993.)

Yoshimoto, T. et al. 1983. "Flavonoids: Potent inhibitors of arachidonate-5-lipoxygenase." *Biochemical Biophysiolgical Research Communication* 116: 612-18.

Chapter 11
Infectious Diseases and Immunity

Baum, M. et al. 1994. "Inadequate dietary intake and altered nutrition status in early HIV-1 infection." *Nutrition* 10: 16-20.

Bendich, A. 1992. "Vitamins and immunity." *Journal of Nutrition* 122: 601-3.

Bliznakov, E. G., and G. L. Hunt. *The Miracle Nutrient: Coenzyme Q_{10}* (New York: Bantam, 1986.)

Bogden, J. D. 1995. Micronutrient nutrition and immunity: Part 2." *Nutrition Report* 9: 16-17.

Bouic, P. J. D. et al. 1995. "Beta-sitosterol and beta-sitosterol glucoside stimulate peripheral blood lymphocyte proliferation: Implications for their use as an immunomodulatory vitamin combination." *International Journal of Immunopharmacology* 18: 693-700.

——. 1997. "Immunomodulation in HIV/AIDS: The Tygerberg/Stellenbosch University experience." *AIDS Bulletin* 6(3).

Clerici, M. et al. 1994. "An immunoendocrinological hypothesis of HIV infection." *Lancet* 343: 1552-53.

Clerici, M., and G. M. Shearer. 1993. A T_H1 to T_H2 switch is a critical step in the etiology of HIV infection." *Immunology Today* 14: 107-11.

Coodley, G. O. et al. 1993. "Micronutrient concentrations in the HIV wasting syndrome." *AIDS Bulletin* 7: 1595-1600.

Coutsoudis, A. et al. 1995. "The effects of vitamin A supplementaion on the morbidity of children born to HIV-infected women." *American Journal of Public Health* 85: 1076-81.

Daynes, R. A. et al. 1993. "Altered regulation of IL-6 production with normal aging." *The Journal of Immunology* 150: 5219-30.

Feinberg, M. B., and W. C. Greene. 1991. "Molecular insights into human immunodeficiency virus type 1 infection." *New England Journal of Medicine* 324(5): 308-17.

Folkers, K. 1988. "Biochemical deficiencies of coenzyme Q_{10} in HIV-infection and exploratory treatment." *Biochemical and Biophysical Research Communications* 153:8 88-96.

Gaby, A. R. 1996. "The role of coenzyme Q_{10} in clinical medicine." *Alternative Medicine Review* 1: 12.

Horowitz, L. G. *Emerging Viruses, AIDS & Ebola, Nature, Accident or Intentional?* (Massachusetts: Tetrahedron Publishing Group, 1997.)

Kalimi, M. et al. 1994. "Anti-glucocorticoid effects of dehydroepiandrosterone (DHEA)." *Molecular and Cellular Biochemistry* 131: 99-104.

Kauffmann, S. H. E. 1993. "Immunity to intracellular bacteria." *Annual Review of Immunology* 11: 129-63.

Kidd, P. M., and W. Huber. *Living With the AIDS Virus: A Strategy for Long-Term Survival.* (California: HK Biomedical, 1990.)

Kimura, M., S. Tanaka, Y. Yamada et al. 1998. "Dehydroepiandrosterone decreases serum tumor necrosis factor-alpha and restores insulin sensitivity: Independent effect from secondary weight reduction in genetically obese Zucker fatty rats." *Endocrinology* 139: 3249-53.

Levy, S. B. *The Antibiotic Paradox: How Miracle Drugs Are Destroying the Miracle.* (Plenum Publishers, 1992.)

Ling, W. H., and P. J. H. Jones. 1995. "Dietary phytosterols: A review of metabolism, benefits and side effects." *Life Sciences* 57: 195-206.

Lockwood, K. et al. 1994. "Partial and complete regression of breast cancer in patients in relation to dosage of coenzyme Q_{10}." *Biochemical and Biophysical Research Communication* 199(3): 1504-8.

Mackenzie, G. et al. 1987. "Inflammatory response to parasites." *Parasitology* 94: 9-10.

Mims, C. A. *The Pathogenesis of Infectious Disease.* (Academic Press, 1987.)

Mulder, J. W. et al. 1992. DHEA as a predictor for progression to AIDS in asymptomatic HIV-infected men." *Journal of Infectious Disease* 165: 413-18.

Regelson, W., R. Loria, and M. Kalimi. 1994. "Dehydroepiandrosterone (DHEA)— the "Mother Steroid." *Annals New York Academy of Science* 121: 553-63.

Rosenbaum, M., and M. Susser. *Solving the Puzzle of Chronic Fatigue Syndrome.* (Tacoma, Washington: Life Sciences Press, 1992.)

Roy, M. et al. 1994. "Supplementation with selenium and human immune cell functions. I. Effect on Lymphocyte Proliferation and Interleukin 2 Receptor Expression." *Biological Trace Element Research* 41: 103-14.

Paul, W. E. 1993. "Infectious diseases and the immune system." *Scientific America* (Sept): 90-97.

Sher, A. and R. L. Coffman. 1992. "Regulation of immunity to parasites by T cells and T cell-derived cytokines." *Annual Review of Immunology* 10: 385-409.

Swab, J. H. "Suppression of the immune response by microorganism." *Bacteriol Review* 39: 121.

Wallace, D. J. et al. 1990. "Fibromyalgia, cytokines, fatigue syndromes and immune regulation." In *Advances in Pain Research and Therapy.* J. R. Fricton and E. Awad. Raven Press. 17: 227-87.

Weiss, R. A. 1993. How Does HIV Cause AIDS? *Science* 260: 1273-79.

Chapter 12
Stress, Exercise, and Immunity

Ben-Nathan, D., et al. 1991. "Protection by dehydroepiandrosterone in mice infected with viral encephalitis." *Archives of Virology* 120: 263-71.

Birkenhager-Gillesse, E. G. et al. 1994. "Dehydroepiandrosterone sulphate (DHEAS) in the oldest old, aged 85 and over." *Annals of the New York Academy of Science* 719: 543-52.

Bouic, P. J. D. et al. 1996. Beta-sitosterol and beta-sitosterol glucoside stimulate human peripheral blood lymphocyte proliferation: Implications for their use as an immunomodulatory vitamin combination." *International Journal of Immunopharmacology* 18: 693-700.

Camus, G. et al. 1994. "Are similar inflammatory factors involved in strenuous exercise and sepsis?" *Intensive Care Medicine* 20: 602-10.

Clerici, M., and G. M. Shearer. 1994. The T_H1-T_H2 hypothesis of HIV infection, new insights." *Immunology Today* 15: 575-81.

Cohen, S. et al. 1991. "Psychological stress and susceptibility to the common cold." *New England Journal of Medicine* 325: 606-12.

Cousins, N. *Anatomy of an Illness.* (New York, W.W. Norton, 1979.)

Dhabhar, F. S. et al. 1995. "Effects of stress on immune cell distribution: Dynamics and hormonal mechanisms." *Journal of Immunology* 154: 5511-27.

Dillon, K. M. et al. 1986. "Positive emotional states and enhancement of the immune system." *International Journal of Psychiatry in Medicine* 15: 13-17.

Gloria, R. M., W. Regelson, and D. A. Padget. "Immune response facilitation and resistance to viral and bacterial infections with DHEA." In *The Biological Role of Dehydroepiandrosterone (DHEA)*, M. Kalimi and W. Regelson. (New York: Walter de Gruyter, 1990.)

Hoffman-Goetz, L., and B. K. Pedersen. "Exercise and the immune system: A model of the stress response." *Immunology Today* 15: 382-87.

Kalimi, M. et al. 1994. Anti-glucocorticoid effects of dehydroepiandrosterone (DHEA)." *Molecular and Cellular Biochemistry* 131: 99-104.

Kalokerinos, A. *Every Second Child.* (New Canaan, Connecticut: Keats Publishing, 1981.)

Kasl, S. V. et al. 1979. Psychosocial risk factors in the development of infectious mononucleosis." *Psychosomatic Medicine* 41: 445-66.

McKay, D. A. "Stress, illness and the physician." *Archives of Family Medicine* 4: 497-98.

Medman, M. E. et al. 1989. "Low sulpho-conjugated steroid hormone levels in systemic lupus erythematosus (SLE)." *Clin. Exp. Rheumatology* 7: 583-88.

Newsholme, E. A. 1994. "Biochemical mechanisms to explain immunosuppression in well-trained and overtrained athletes." *International Journal of Sports Medicine* 15: 142-47.

Nieman, D. C. 1994. "Exercise, infection and immunity." *International Journal of Sports Medicine* 15: 131-41.

———. 1994. "Exercise, upper respiratory tract infections, and the immune system." *Medicine and Science in Sports and Exercise* 26: 128-39.

Northoff H., C. Weinstock, and A. Berg. 1994. "The cytokine response to strenuous exercise." *International Journal of Sports Medicine* 15: 167-71.

Orentreich, N. J. et al. 1987. "Age changes and sex differences in serum dehydroepiandrosterone sulfate concentrations throughout adulthood." *Journal of Clinical Endocrinological Metabolism* 59: 551-55.

Padgett, D. A. and R. M. Loria. 1994. "In vitro potentiation of lymphocyte activation by dehydroepiandrosterone, androstenediol, and androstenetriol." *Journal Immunology* 153: 1544-51.

Pennebaker, J. W. et al. 1977. "Lack of control as a determinant of perceived physical symptoms." *Journal of Personal Social Psychology* 35(3): 167-74.

Peters, E. M. et al. 1993. "Vitamin C supplementation reduces the incidence of post race symptoms of upper respiratory-tract infection in ultramarathon runners." *American Journal of Clinical Nutrition* 57: 170-74.

Regelson, W., R. Loria, and M. Kalimi. 1994. "Dehydroepiandrosterone (DHEA)—the mother steroid." *Annals New York Academy of Sciences* 121: 553-63.

Reichert, R. *Kava kava.* (New Canaan, Connecticut: Keats Publishing, 1998.)

Rook, G. A. W. et al. 1994. "Hormones, peripherally activated prohormones, and the regulation of the T_H1/T_H2 balance." *Immunology Today* 15: 301-3.

Sachs, B. C. Coping with stress. *Stress Medicine* 7: 61-63.

Shepard, R. J., and P. N. Shek. 1994. "Infectious diseases in athletes: New interest for an old problem." *Journal of Sports Medicine and Physical Fitness* 34: 11-22.

Sparling, P. B., D. C. Nieman, and P. J. O'Connor. 1993. "Selected scientific aspects of marathon racing. An update on fluid replacement, immune function, psychological factors and the gender difference." *Sports Medicine* 15: 116-32.

Index

Flaxseed oil, 60, 61, 66, 71, 150, 213, 215
Folkers, K., 34
Food processing, 42
Food sources, 31
    beta-carotene, 44
    carotenoids, 44
    coenzyme Q_{10}, 34–35
    DHA, 141
    EPA, 141
    essential fats, 61
    essential fatty acids, 66
    fiber, 77–78
    flavonoids, 44
    glutathione, 36
    indoles, 53
    isoflavones, 52
    lignans, 52, 65
    lycopene, 44
    magnesium, 38
    phytoestrogens, 51–52
    phytonutrients, 42–43
    protein, 78–79
    saturated fats, 62
    selenium, 30
    sterols, 47–51, 53, 60
    vitamin A, 34
    vitamin B_6, 37
    vitamin C, 33
    zinc, 29
Food-labeling regulations, 63
Foods
    acid/alkaline, 79–81
    barbecued, 65
    blackened, 65
    cholesterol-free, 60, 63
    cooking oils, 65
    cruciferous vegetables, 69
    deep-frying, 65
    fiber, 77–78
    fruits. See Fruits
    genetically engineered, 67
    hydrogenated, 64
    immune system cure, 67–68
    organic, 25, 58
    overeating, 74–75
    red meat, 65
    refined foods, 82
    seeds and nuts, 66
    vegetables. See Vegetables
    in whole form, 57
Fortification, 25
Foster, Harold, 29
Fountain of youth, 30
Foxglove, 4
Free radicals, 26–27, 65, 68–69

Freezing, 42
Fruits, 71–73, 104
    see also Phytonutrients

G
Gamma linolenic acid, 140, 150–151
Garlic, 68–69
Genetically engineered foods, 67
Genistein. See Phytoestrogens
Gerson, Max, 6
Gibson, Stewart, 188–189
Gingko biloba, 51
Ginseng, 52, 104–105
Glucosamine sulphate, 148–149
Glutathione, 29–30, 35–36, 53–54, 141–142
Granulocytes, 11
Green Alive, 78
Green drinks, 78, 216
Green tea, 83
GREENS+, 78
Guided imagery, 93

H
Harpagophytum procumbens, 51
Harzol, 118
Healing spas, 222
Healthy Living Guide, 153
Healthy Pleasures, 90
Heart attacks, 199
Heavy metal poisoning, 132–134
Helper T-cells. See T-cells
Hepatitis
    hepatitis A, 179, 186
    hepatitis B, 31, 179, 186–187
    hepatitis C, 187
    medical therapies, 187–188
    resources, 223
    Sterinol, 188–189
    vitamin C, 189
Heredity, 125–126, 168
Hesperidin, 43
Histamine, 21, 162
HIV, 4, 10, 179
    DHEA, 184–185
    disease progression, 35, 180–181
    resources, 217–219
    and selenium, 30
    statistics, 181
    and Sterinol, 47, 106, 182–184
    T-cells, 180, 182
    vitamin B_6, 37
    vitamin C, 185
    see also AIDS
Hives, 166–167
Hoffer, Abram, 31, 56